Praise for *High Performance Vision*

"The philosophy that you need"

"Dr. Don Teig's program proves
that you need to be visually fit, not ju
want to gain a competitive edge. The
throughout these pages will put you
your game if you take the time and effo

part of your training routine. I really appreciate Don's skill and technological knowledge, as well as his sincere commitment to keeping the eyes healthy. I am confident this book will help you in your quest for excellence."

–Joe Torre
National Baseball Hall of Famer (2014)
Executive Vice President of Baseball Operations, Major League Baseball

"The recognized pioneer in this field"

"Maximizing my vision and my approach to visualizing success as a goaltender was always a high priority in my career. Dr. Teig is the recognized pioneer in this field. His knowledge and approach to training my eyes helped me to achieve my goals as a professional athlete."

–John Vanbiesbrouck
US Hockey Hall of Fame Goaltender

"Dr. Teig has been a leader in this technology"

"The improvement of efficient vision skills over the years has had a huge impact on major league baseball, especially the hitters. Dr. Teig has been a leader in this technology ever since I was a player in the seventies, when he worked with me to improve my vision skills."

–Chris Chambliss
Former Major League All-Star First Baseman

"How to get the most out of my vision"

"Dr. Don Teig's program proves the philosophy
that you need to be visually fit, not just physically fit,
if you want to gain a competitive edge. The information
discussed throughout these pages will put you on track to
improve your game if you take the time and effort to make
these drills part of your training routine. I really appreciate
Don's skill and technological knowledge, as well as his sincere
commitment to keeping the eyes healthy. I am confident this
book will help you in your quest for excellence."

–Paula Creamer
LPGA Champion Golfer

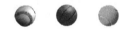

"Will help anyone looking for that edge"

"Every professional team or athlete is in a constant search
to improve performance. Sports vision is a vital avenue
in this search. Don Teig has been passionate about the
relationship between vision and performance for forty years.
He has worked with many different athletes in various sports.
This book will help anyone looking for that edge."

–Steve Donohue
Head Athletic Trainer
New York Yankees

"A must-read"

"This book is a must-read for any professional in the
field of player improvement. Dr. Teig is a visionary and
pioneer in the discipline of vision and neuromuscular testing
and training. The future of athletic development will be
in the hands of the vision-training coach as much as
the strength and fitness coach. This is truly cutting
edge for the amateur or professional athlete."

–Mike Saunders
Former NY Knicks Head Medical Trainer
NBA Trainer of the Year.

HIGH
PERFORMANCE
VISION

HOW TO IMPROVE YOUR VISUAL ACUITY, HONE YOUR MOTOR SKILLS & UP YOUR GAME

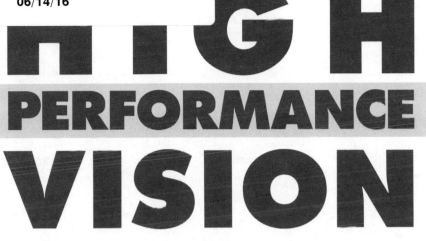

HIGH PERFORMANCE VISION

HOW TO IMPROVE YOUR VISUAL ACUITY, HONE YOUR MOTOR SKILLS & UP YOUR GAME

DR. DONALD S. TEIG

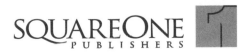

SQUAREONE
PUBLISHERS

COVER DESIGNER: Jeannie Tudor
EDITOR: Michael Weatherhead
TYPESETTER: Gary A. Rosenberg

The information and advice contained in this book are based upon the research and the personal and professional experiences of the author. They are not intended as a substitute for consulting with a health care professional. The publisher and author are not responsible for any adverse effects or consequences resulting from the use of any of the suggestions, preparations, or procedures discussed in this book. All matters pertaining to your physical health should be supervised by a health care professional. It is a sign of wisdom, not cowardice, to seek a second or third opinion.

Square One Publishers
115 Herricks Road   516-535-2010 • 877-900-BOOK
Garden City Park, NY 1104   www.squareonepublishers.com

Library of Congress Cataloging-in-Publication Data
Teig, Donald S.
  High performance vision / Dr. Donald S. Teig.
    pages cm
  ISBN 978-0-7570-0399-8
  1. Visual training. 2. Depth perception. 3. Eye—Care and hygiene.
4. Self-care, Health. I. Title.
  RE960.T45 2015
  612.8'4—dc23

                                            2015020846

Printed in the United States of America

10   9   8   7   6   5   4   3   2   1

Contents

Acknowledgments

Presenting in book form the knowledge I have gained over my many years of working with athletes was a truly daunting task. I will forever be grateful to my publisher, Rudy Shur, for constantly encouraging me to share my expertise with the athlete population in this way. I want to express my appreciation to my editor, Michael Weatherhead, for keeping me on the straight and narrow as I organized my thoughts to create a book that would motivate all athletes to go for the gold.

Special thanks go out to Dr. John Diamond—world-renowned expert in holistic medicine, musician extraordinaire, and true gentleman—for urging me to write this book so that athletes of all levels of proficiency could achieve their competitive goals by getting the most out of their eyes. Of course, I would be remiss in not mentioning the many athletes, coaches, trainers, and friends who helped lay the groundwork for me to excel in a specialty that has always been near and dear to my heart. Such mentors as Pat Riley, Joe Torre, Steve Donohue, Mike Saunders, Bucky Dent, Patrick Ewing, Gene Monahan, Dave Smith, Fran Healy, Mike Keenan, and Roger Nielson, to name only a few, all played roles in my success. There were so many fine people alongside me on my journey that I am certain I am unintentionally omitting a few who guided me along the way.

Perhaps the greatest cheerleader has been my wife, Joyce, who has put up with my many hours of dedication to this field while always providing me with encouragement and a sounding board for my thoughts. Thanks to her, the hills and valleys along my path have not seemed too high or too wide to traverse. What should drive a man most is his family, and the love I share with my son, Jason, and my daughter, Lori, make me appreciate how important family is to all that we do and accomplish in our lives. After all, the rest of this is just a game!

Foreword

I was introduced to Dr. Teig and his pioneering approach to vision during my time as a New York Yankee over forty years ago. Even back then, every player was looking for a way to gain a competitive edge, and it made complete sense to me that improving my eyesight was the way to go if I truly wanted to raise the level of my game. Throughout my playing and coaching careers, I have often included Dr. Teig's eye exercises and visualization methods as part of my training regimen, as well as the training regimens of players under my guidance at the "Bucky Dent Baseball Academy" in Delray Beach, Florida. Over the years, I have enjoyed many conversations with Dr. Teig about the game we both love, and about how optimizing eyesight can mean the difference between being a good athlete and an elite athlete. Understandably, when my son Cody began his professional baseball career, a visit to Dr. Teig's clinic was high on his list of priorities.

I urge every athlete, coach, and sports parent to read *High Performance Vision* from cover to cover and digest all the pearls of wisdom Dr. Teig has to offer. His innovative approach to eyesight undoubtedly played a major role in my athletic career, and it can in yours as well.

Bucky Dent
Starting shortstop, New York Yankees (1977–1982)
MLB World Series MVP (1978)
Three-time MLB All-Star
Manager, New York Yankees (1989–1990)

Preface

I wrote this book to pass along the knowledge I have gained over a forty-year career dedicated to enhancing the visual motor skills of athletes. My goal remains simple: to help you improve your game. More broadly, I would like to help you feel the enjoyment that comes with overcoming the obstacles standing in the way of your athletic success. I have been fortunate to be privy to the knowledge of a number of experts over the course of my career, from athletes and coaches to athletic trainers and medical colleagues. Along with my own observations and hands-on experience, I have distilled and adapted this knowledge into the high performance vision program.

It has always seemed obvious to me that success in athletics must begin with the best possible sense of vision. And by vision I do not mean simply eyesight, which may be defined as the ability to see the world. Vision is an acquired skill that is guided by the way we interpret what we see. For example, if you had never seen a cow, you would still have the eyesight to recognize a strange animal in your path if a cow were to walk in front of you. It is only through learning and experience, however, that you would be able to label this animal a cow.

I intend to guide you through the world of vision in a concise, understandable manner, so that you may use your most precious sense to improve the way you play sports. It will take practice and dedication, but you will see the difference high performance vision training can bring.

In an effort to avoid awkward phrasing within sentences, it is our publishing style to alternate the use of male and female pronouns according to chapter. Therefore, when referring to a "third-person" adult, child, healthcare provider, or caregiver, odd-numbered chapters will use female pronouns, while even-numbered chapters will use male, to give acknowledgment to people of both genders.

HIGH PERFORMANCE VISION

Introduction

To paraphrase boxing legend Muhammed Ali, "Float like a butterfly, sting like a bee, your hands can't hit what your eyes can't see!" Ali may have been talking about the speed of his legs, but he unintentionally made a more important point about the role of vision in athletics. The fact is that, when it comes to sports, you are only as good as your eyes. And just as exercise and practice can increase your strength and speed, so may high performance vision training enhance your visual system.

It's your eyes that alert and activate your motor system so that you can react with split-second timing. But there's more to keeping your eyes on an object than merely looking at it, no matter how hard you concentrate. You have to see not only where the object is but also where it is going, how fast it is traveling, and how much spin it has on it. If it sounds difficult, that's because it is. Some people play sports for years and never quite get the most out of their eyes. That's a shame because, in most cases, you can improve your visual system and actually train yourself to see better by means of a fairly simple program known as high performance vision training. While you may do this training at a specialized clinic, you may also practice many high performance vision exercises on the playing field and in the privacy of your own home, as you will discover.

In over thirty years of evaluating and training the visual skills of athletes, I have had the privilege of improving the on-field performance of a wide variety of competitors, including little leaguers, weekend warriors, and some of the finest athletes in the world. Who could have predicted that the equipment and eye exercises I developed with the help of engineers, coaches, athletic trainers, and the very athletes I sought to help would have evolved into a specialty program that has taken me all over the world? Until now, I have carefully shared my knowledge only with the athletes who have trained with me. My intent now is to share this program with you.

Part One begins at the beginning and asks you to set goals. They can be general. For example, "I want to improve my overall athletic performance by making my eyes more efficient." They can also be targeted to specific needs. For example, "I want to reduce my number of strokes during eighteen holes of golf to thirty-five or less."

You'll then learn the basic biology of vision to get a better understanding of how the human eye actually takes in light and sends data to the brain to be processed into images. The pros and cons of various corrective options, including glasses, contact lenses, and Lasik, will also be reviewed. After this tutorial, you'll find a list of the most common eye problems, including injuries and the specific sport with which each is associated. You'll become familiar with the symptoms of these conditions and the treatments typically administered to alleviate them. Finally, you'll see how to measure your visual skills as you consider a proper training program.

Part Two starts by examining the role of vision in sports and explains the parameters within which a doctor determines a patient's overall vision. Next, you'll dive into high performance vision training in earnest as this book gives you a comprehensive list of exercises that will help you hone your visual system to its peak potential, whether in a clinical setting, on the field, or from the comfort of your own home. You'll also get detailed sport-specific drills and exercises, which are sure to provide you with an even sharper edge in your chosen activity. By taking advantage of all the high performance vision tools at your disposal, you'll be truly amazed by the degree to which your game will improve.

All athletes want to be in "the zone" as often as possible during competition. Most find getting there an elusive and daunting task. No matter how much you practice, you may feel as though you've hit a wall in terms of performance. High performance vision training was designed to break down this wall. After all, 80 percent of all sensory information to the brain comes through the eyes. Use this book as a guide and get yourself to the place beyond the wall.

PART ONE

Getting Started

High performance vision training can be the element that transforms a good athlete into an exceptional athlete. Vision involves many subtle and sophisticated links between the eyes, brain, and muscles. The stamina, flexibility, and fine-tuning of your visual system can provide you with the split-second timing you need to excel in competition. But what does "high performance vision" actually mean? It is a term that refers to the distinction between the ability to see clearly and the ability to see even better than that. It is defined by a visual system that is beyond what most would consider the norm. Training your eyes through the use of a specific set of eye exercises can take you to a level of athletic achievement you may not have thought possible.

1.

Setting Your Goals

It has been written that you stand a better chance of achieving what you want in life if you define your goals clearly and put them in writing. Your primary goal might be something like, "I want to become a better hitter," or, "I want to be the best free-throw shooter on the team," or, "I want to be first-string quarterback for the varsity team." Your primary goal can be whatever you want it to be. Don't be afraid to think big. Of course, achieving your primary goal will depend on many factors. Perhaps more than any other factor, hard work represents the ultimate key to achieving your goal. Having the right mindset to succeed can also go a long way. Yogi Berra, the great baseball catcher and philosopher, said it best in his inimitable manner. According to Yogi, "Baseball is 90 percent mental and the other half is physical."

There is also something to be said for raw talent, which is often genetically predetermined. For example, it certainly helps to grow to seven feet tall if you want to excel in basketball. Finally, as with many things in life, it doesn't hurt to be lucky! There's something to be said for being in the right place at the right time. All things being considered, however, the best way to travel down the road towards your goal (or goals) is to be driven. You need to chase the proverbial carrot. But in your case, you can reach it if you put in the work.

Once you've established your primary goal, your next step will be to break down that goal into its components. How are you going to become the player you want to be? Is it through practice, studying top players, going to camps, or working with specialized instructors? Whatever the case may be, high performance vision will most definitely play a large role in the successful completion of your objective.

At this point, you simply need to begin by stating your primary goal.

My primary goal is:

_____

_____

_____

In order to achieve this goal, I plan to work in these areas:

_____

_____

_____

_____

_____

Now that you have stated the destination at which you wish to arrive on your high performance vision journey and clarified how you plan on getting there, it's time to get to the details of your game plan.

HIGH PERFORMANCE VISION GOALS

So, what would you like to get out of a program of high performance vision training? Certainly the aspirations of a hockey goaltender are going to differ from those of a golfer. Perhaps you play more than one sport. Maybe you play more than one position in a given sport. Each position or sport may have its own requirement. While some requirements may be common to a number of positions (a shortstop and first baseman may both want to develop the skills needed to become better hitters), some will be different. The glue that keeps these goals together is one very critical common bond. Simply put, it is getting the most out of your most valuable asset: your eyes.

Write down some of the sport-specific or position-specific goals you have for high performance vision training. This may not be an easy task, especially if you are new to this concept. The following examples may be helpful:

- You'd like to improve your ability to hold your eyes steady when shooting a basketball.

- You'd like to identify the movement of the ball sooner when batting.

- You'd like to see all your receivers during a passing play.

- You'd like to be able to read the greens better when putting.

Now list your goals as they relate to vision improvement:

_____

_____

_____

_____

_____

_____

SPORT-SPECIFIC QUESTIONNAIRE

Here are some specific sports-related vision questions that should be answered before you embark on your high performance vision program. By honestly answering these questions to the best of your ability, you will get a better understanding of the role your eyes will play in your quest for excellence in your chosen sport. Before starting your high performance vision program, the content of these questions and answers will guide you, as well as any trained professional, to consider all the ways in which your vision can help you achieve your athletic goals. These are straightforward questions designed to enable you and your trainer or coach to begin on the right track.

1. **Do you ever experience blurred vision?**　　　　　　　Y__ N__

   If yes, where?　Far distance ____　Near distance ___

   How often? _____

   While competing?　**Y__ N__**　If yes, describe: _____

   _____

2. **Do you ever see double?**　　　　　　　　　　　　Y__ N__

   If yes, where?　Far distance ____　Near distance ___

   How often? _____

   While competing? **Y__ N__**　If yes, how often? _____

   _____

3. **Do you ever have difficulty "keeping your eye"
   on a moving object?**　　　　　　　　　　　　　Y__ N__

   If yes, describe: _____

   _____

4. **Do you notice variations in your performance during an event?** Y__ N__

   If yes, describe: _____

   _____

10

5. **Do you notice variations in your performance over a period of time?** Y__ N__

   If yes, describe: _____

   _____

6. **When is your performance most consistent during a sporting event?**

   Early ____   Later ____   Throughout ____

7. **Is performance consistent during critical competition situations?** Y__ N__

   Explain: _____

   _____

8. **Where applicable, is your performance the same at night as it is during the day?** Y__ N__

9. **Do you experience loss of concentration during events?** Y__ N__

   If yes, describe: _____

   _____

10. **Have you been experiencing any visual difficulties?** Y__ N__

    If yes, describe: _____

    _____

11. **Have you ever participated in any form of vision training?** Y__ N__

    If yes, describe: _____

    _____

12. **If you have had previous vision training, do you feel it was successful?** Y__ N__

    If yes, explain: _____

    _____

13. **Do you wear eyeglasses?**   Y__ N__

   If yes, why do you wear eyeglasses?

   Distance___ Near___ Both___

14. **Do you presently wear contact lenses?**   Y__ N__

   If yes, which type?

   Soft___ Gas-permeable___ Corneal-molding___

15. **Do you wear contact lenses while competing?**   Y__ N__

16. **Are you experiencing any problems with your**
    current lenses?   Y__ N__

   If yes, describe: _____

   _____

17. **Have you undergone LASIK surgery?**   Y__ N__

   If yes, describe outcome: _____

   _____

18. **Please rate the importance of vision in your chosen sport.**

   1 2 3 4 5 6 7 8 9

   (1 = not important; 9 = extremely important.)

19. **Do you use visualization or positive-imagery techniques?**   Y__ N__

   If yes, describe: _____

   _____

Answering these eye-related questions is a crucial step along the right path to high performance vision. You will enhance your visual skill through this program by meeting both general and specific goals.

FINDING THE RIGHT DOCTOR

The sports world has seen an explosion of interest in the area of vision and cognition. Athletes and coaches now recognize the visual system—which triggers the brain to send a message to the muscles and allows the body to perform at its optimum level—as the starting point in athletic training. New technologies have helped to advance the notion that improving vision is the main method by which athletes may attain a competitive edge. Unfortunately, for now, only a handful of medical professionals possess the proper training and expertise to meet the needs of the athletic population. Thankfully, an elite group of professionals armed with expertise in high performance vision training have organized under the banner of high performance vision associates. I am very happy to report that this organization of providers is growing daily and will hopefully include more members throughout the United States and Canada soon. For more information about these professionals, consult the Resources section (see page 141) at the end of this book.

CONCLUSION

Before you begin down the road to high performance vision, it is vital to establish your specific goals, grasp the visual elements common to your chosen sport, and understand how your personality can impact your training and ultimate athletic achievement. If you chose to train with a doctor or coach, there are now doctors and trainers versed in high performance vision techniques who can guide you along your way to better vision and overall athletic success. It is now time to turn your attention to the basics of vision, including the anatomy of the eye and the most common methods used in vision correction.

2.

Vision Basics

I t is often said that the eyes work like a camera. This statement is true to a degree, although it is a gross oversimplification. No camera can match the intricacy with which the eye allows a view of the world. Before you can fully understand how to get the most out of your vision as an athlete, you need to familiarize yourself with the components that make up the structure of the human eye. Once you have done this, you may then determine the best way to implement the most efficient approach to maximize your visual system. This chapter considers both the anatomical components of the eye, which are instrumental to the sense of sight, as well as the psychophysical aspect of vision, which helps the brain interpret the light traveling through the eyes.

ANATOMY OF THE HUMAN EYE

While the eyes are the windows to the soul, they are also the windows to the brain. Light rays travel through the eyes to send a message to the brain, which helps you choose what to do next in any given situation. To explain this in greater detail, sight begins with light rays traveling through the tear film, which coats the front surface of the eyes. The next stop along this path to proper vision is the cornea. This transparent dome floats over a fluid channel called the aqueous humor. This fluid channel sits in what is referred to as the anterior chamber of the eye. The hole in the center of the iris (the structure that gives eyes their color), also known as the pupil, then allows light to pass through the iris, allowing these rays to travel on their way to their ultimate goal of reaching the retina. The light must still, however, travel through the gel-like liquid called the vitreous humor, which comprises almost two-thirds of the inside cavity of the eye globe. Finally, these light rays impact the retinal surface (the photosensitive rods and cones layer) before sending an impulse to the optic nerve, which leaves the eye to stimulate the visual control center of the occipital back lobe of the brain known as the visual cortex. (See Figure 2.1.)

Rods are significantly more plentiful on the retinal surface and are essential for peripheral vision as well as night vision. The less

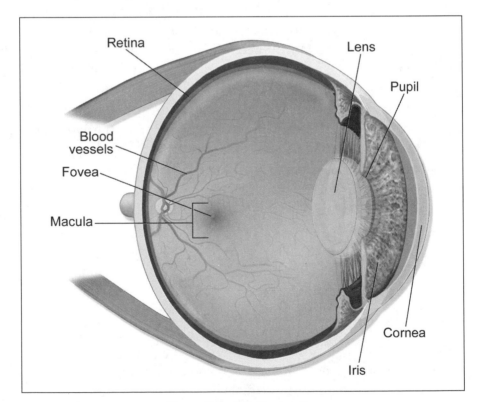

Figure 2.1. The Human Eye

prevalent cones are contained mostly in the macular area of the retina. This pinhead-sized dot is critical for providing crisp, sharp central vision, as well as an appreciation of colors. Ultimately, all this valuable visual information arrives at the brain and alerts the body to react with its neuromuscular system appropriately.

The Human Eye

Until now, this book's description of vision has been limited to the physical path of light through the eye, which ultimately creates a message that travels from the optic nerve to the brain. At this point, we must move beyond this description.

We may all see things essentially the same, but we usually perceive them very differently from each other. Much of this phenomenon can be attributed to exposure to diverse environments during childhood and adolescence. Humans are deeply influenced by their external surroundings and internal emotions, the mixture of which may produce very distinctive ways of seeing the world. Many sports impose tremendous visual demands on the visual system as athletes attempt to excel in their fields.

Consider the very intricate art and science of hitting a baseball. When a major league baseball pitcher throws a ninety-mile-per-hour fastball, the batter has less than half a second to see the pitch, judge its speed and location, decide what to do, and then start to swing. The bat must meet the ball within an eighth of an inch of dead center, and at precisely the right millisecond as the three-inch spinning sphere whizzes by. "It is a superhuman feat that is clearly impossible!" according to Robert Adair, a Yale physicist who has studied the science of baseball.

CORRECTING YOUR BASIC VISION

It never ceases to amaze me that some of the most elite athletes I have had the privilege to work with in my career have not considered the possibility that they could see better by using corrective methods. When you think about it, it's likely that you, as an athlete, may not be aware that you are not seeing as optimally as possible. After all, how can you tell if your sight is even on par with what others are seeing? If you don't investigate, then you don't find out. An amazing case of not knowing is the fact that the great baseball legend, Babe Ruth, who had poor vision in one eye, never had his eyes examined until after his playing days. It was only then that doctors discovered that one eye was significantly weaker than the other. If he was that good with one properly working eye, imagine if he'd had two!

I am the first to admit, however, that athletes can achieve greatness with less-than-efficient eyes. After all, there are a multitude of factors that lead to athletic success. Great genes, great mechanics, hard work, a good attitude, and learning how to compensate for deficiencies all come to mind. But they don't negate the fact that two strong eyes that work together as a team will always be better than two weak eyes that don't. Of course, when it comes to correcting your vision, the debate rages on over which choice is best for athletes. Options include eyeglasses, contact lenses, corneal molding, and LASIK surgery, and the truth is that there is no clear-cut right choice. Much varies by individual as well as the unique demands of each sport.

Eyeglasses

Eyeglasses are the most common corrective option, but they are not the best choice for every sport. For example, they are pretty much a no-no in hockey. They simply fog up on the ice and may not fit comfortably under a visor. On the other hand, they can be perfectly fine for trap shooters. Shooters are typically required to wear specially designed shooting glasses, so why not use a prescription pair, if necessary?

As an athlete, you need to be aware of the latest technology in corrective lenses available. The most efficient corrective lenses today provide such things as superior optics, aberration (distortion) control, glare treatment, sport-specific tints, light weight, and exceptional protection from injury.

You may be asking what lens aberrations are. These are a variety of distortions that influence an athlete's ability to see objects with uncompromising detail. They include components of optics such as spherical aberration, coma, and trefoil. While the science of this issue is beyond the scope of this book, suffice it to say that lenses can minimize these distortions and allow you to see more clearly and with better contrast.

Sport-specific tints on lenses can impact decision-making during competition. All sunglass lenses are tinted to cut down on overall brightness and enhance terrain definition, but your choice of tint color can affect your vision by influencing how much visible light reaches your eyes and how well you see other colors and interpret contrast. If you'd like to try tinted lenses, be sure to choose the right tint for your sport, taking playing conditions into consideration.

Vermilion Lenses

Vermilion-tinted, or rose-colored, glasses really do make the world seem brighter. They provide excellent clarity in low light and enhance contrast. As a result, they are great for skiing and snowboarding in cloudy conditions. They also enhance the visibility of objects against blue and green backgrounds, which makes them ideal for trap shooting.

Brown, Gray, or Green Lenses

Lenses that are brown, gray, or green do an outstanding job of reducing glare without distorting appreciation of different colors. These lenses are particularly effective in moderately bright to very bright conditions.

Yellow, Gold, or Amber Lenses

Lenses that are yellow, gold, or amber (previously known as "Calichrome") provide some brightness protection but are more effective in moderately bright to low-level light conditions. They provide strong depth perception, which makes them perfect for skiing, snowboarding, and other snow sports. They also enhance the ability to appreciate detail in flatly lighted conditions. These lenses work very efficiently under hazy lighting conditions and perform especially well during dawn and dusk.

Mirrored Lenses

Mirror-coated lenses refer to a reflective film applied to the outside surface of sunglass lenses. Mirrored lenses reduce glare by reflecting much of the light that hits the lens. The downside is that the mirror coating makes objects appear darker than they are, so lighter tints are often used to compensate for this fact. These lenses are good at cutting glare on a bright sunny day, so they are beneficial to people who play outfield or fish off a boat.

Photochromic Lenses

These lenses automatically adjust to changing light intensities to protect you in a wider range of conditions. They get darker (to block more light) on bright days and lighter when conditions grow dark. If you purchase photochromic lenses you should be aware that the photochromic process takes longer to work in cold conditions, and it doesn't work at all when driving a car (UVB rays do not penetrate the windshield).

Polarized Lenses

Polarization is of exceptional benefit if you are active in water sports or are especially sensitive to glare. When light reflects off flat surfaces, such as a lake, the light waves align in horizontal patterns, creating intense glare. The filters in polarized lenses block these horizontal light waves, substantially reducing blinding glare and its resulting eyestrain. The newest high-end technology combines the polarizing filter with the lens material itself while the latter is still in liquid form. This allows the filter and lens to bond without use of adhesives, which helps maintain an exceptionally high optical quality.

UV Protection

Ultraviolet (UV) rays from the sun can damage your eyes by contributing to cataract, macular degeneration, and growths on the eye, including cancerous melanomas. UVB rays are the main concern for the eyes. According to the American Academy of Optometry, "Long-term exposure to ultraviolet (UV) radiation in sunlight is linked to eye disease. UVB radiation is considered more dangerous to eyes and skin than UVA radiation." UVA rays are the type most absorbed by the eyes, so, while they pose far less concern than UVB rays, doctors recommend avoiding them. UVC rays, of course, are not a concern, as they are blocked by the atmosphere.

UV protection information should be printed on the hangtag or price sticker of any pair of sunglasses you buy, no matter where you buy them. If it isn't, find a different pair. Also keep in mind that cheap tinted sunglasses with limited UV protection can actually do more harm than good, as they cause your pupils to open up wider, leaving your lens even more vulnerable to UV rays. Children's eyes are especially vulnerable to UV light, since they don't have the same level of natural protection as those of adults.

Visible Light Transmission (VLT)

The amount of light that reaches your eyes through your lenses is called "visible light transmission" (VLT). Measured as a percentage, VLT is affected by the color and thickness of your lenses, the material of these lenses, and the coatings they may have on them.

All-purpose sunglasses have a VLT of around 15 to 25 percent. Aim for glasses somewhere in this range if you need a pair for everyday use or basic recreational activities. Glacier glasses (special sunglasses designed specifically to protect eyes from the intense light at high altitudes) have a VLT of around 4 to 10 percent. Most glacier glasses also have shields to protect eyes from light coming in from the sides of the lenses. Because of their low percentage of light transmission, glacier glasses should not be used for driving or any other everyday activities.

Polycarbonate Lenses

The material used in the lenses of your sunglasses will affect their clarity, weight, durability, and cost. Polycarbonate lenses have excellent impact resistance and very good optical clarity. They are also affordable, lightweight, and low bulk. Unfortunately, they are less scratch resistant than glass or NXT polyurethane and offer slightly less optical clarity than these other options.

Polycarbonate was developed in the 1970s for aerospace applications and is currently used for the helmet visors of astronauts and for windshields on space shuttles. Eyeglass lenses made of polycarbonate were introduced in the early 1980s in response to a demand for lightweight, impact-resistant lenses. Since then, polycarbonate lenses have become the standard for safety glasses, sports goggles, and children's eyewear. Because they are less likely to fracture than regular plastic lenses, polycarbonate lenses are also a good choice for rimless eyewear designs, in which lenses are attached to frame components with drill mountings.

Most other plastic lenses are made from a cast-molding process, in which a liquid plastic material is baked for long periods in lens forms, solidifying the liquid plastic to create a lens.

Polycarbonate is a thermoplastic that starts as a solid material in the form of small pellets. In a lens manufacturing process called injection molding, these pellets are heated until they melt. The liquid polycarbonate is then rapidly injected into lens molds, compressed under high pressure, and cooled to form a finished lens product in a matter of minutes.

NXT Polyurethane Lenses

While they may be expensive, NXT polyurethane lenses offer superior impact resistance, excellent optical clarity, great flexibility, and a light weight. Like polycarbonate lenses, they are suitable for safety applications, sportswear, and children's eyewear. NXT polyurethane lenses, sold under the brand name Trivex, are made via a cast-molding process similar to the way in which regular plastic lenses are processed, which gives them crisper optics than lenses made by injection-molding.

Contact Lenses

Just as eyeglasses should be avoided in certain sports, contact lenses may be a somewhat risky choice in others, including wrestling, in which they may become dislodged when any move is applied to the head. Yet contacts are a blessing in golf, tennis, basketball, soccer, and football, just to name a few popular sports in which they are the best option.

When looking into the possibility of wearing contact lenses, much time and consideration should be given to issues such as lens material, lens diameter, water content, and lens stability and positioning. As an athlete, your first decision, perhaps, should be whether to wear contact lenses at all when you could opt for eyeglasses instead. Certainly, some of the more physically dangerous sports demand the use of contact lenses. On the other hand, extremely mild refractive errors may be better served by wearing eyeglasses. The following are the main issues to consider when thinking about getting contact lenses.

Contrast Sensitivity

It's not enough for a budding superstar to experience 20/20 vision while competing. Contrast sensitivity, or the ability to appreciate fine detail, takes eyesight to another level. What separates the average young athlete from the future Hall of Famer is the uncanny talent of that athlete to discriminate between subtleties in vision precisely, such as the rotation of the stitches on a baseball or the location and depth of moguls in skiing. Some contact lenses achieve this goal thanks to their unique resistance to protein buildup. Lens materials must either be resistant to this buildup of debris, easily cleaned, or replaced frequently enough to prevent clouding, which would impair visual judgment and overall athletic performance.

No-Feel Comfort

An athlete cannot afford the distraction of a scratchy contact lens on the eye while in the heat of competition. How often are the terms "focus" and "in the zone" spoken when athletes describe what makes the difference in achieving a competitive edge? An uncomfortable contact lens sets both concepts out of reach. One-day disposable lens designs are often a good choice in regard to comfort, as each day they are brand new.

Convenience

Athletes lead a hectic lifestyle. There is barely time to get everything accomplished in a given day. They are constantly practicing, playing, and traveling. To make it much more likely for athletes to comply with proper contact-lens care, the cleansing routine must be quick and easy.

Stability and Durability

Athletes play rough. Their lenses need to be tough. The lens polymer must be durable enough to withstand aggressive handling in the heat of battle. They must also be stable in their positioning on the eye. Lenses such as the Bausch & Lomb PureVision2 HD for Astigmatism and the SynergEyes Duette maintain stability in correcting astigmatism while being durable.

Uncompromising to Corneal Health

It goes without saying that a healthy eye is your highest priority as a wearer of contact lenses. Any lens that will compromise your eye health is a lens you should not wear. Regular follow-up visits to your eyecare professional are essential to maintain the health and safety of your eyes.

Ease of Handling

This rule is simple: Avoid flimsy, difficult-to-handle lenses. Athletes just don't have the time to deal with these materials when the game is on the line.

Optic Zones and Oversized Diameters

Typically, sports contact lenses are fitted with large optic zones and oversized diameters. A lens must stay positioned well, especially in sports that involve rapid movement and a lot of physical contact. A wrestler, for example, most certainly would benefit from a large-diameter lens over a smaller version when attempting to break away from a headlock.

Water Content

Swimmers generally favor large low-water-content lenses. These stay in place better and are less likely to be contaminated by bacteria or chemicals in the pool. Low-water-content lenses can also increase contrast sensitivity.

Astigmatism

Following the advice of a misinformed practitioner, an athlete may wrongly assume he cannot wear contact lenses due to astigmatism. The truth is that a wide variety of soft and rigid lenses address all types of astigmatism.

Corneal Molding

Precision corneal molding is a non-surgical way to reshape the cornea and correct vision problems. This method uses FDA-approved therapeutic contact lenses. Worn during sleep, these lenses adjust the cornea throughout the night, resulting in clear vision throughout the next day. The ability to participate in sports without the restrictions that eyeglasses and contact lenses impose is a very exciting new reality for the competitive athlete of any age. Imagine contact lenses that allow you the freedom to wear absolutely no corrective lenses during your waking hours, not even while you compete in your chosen sport. It's an amazing thought. You could achieve a sharpness of vision without appliances or other encumbrances on your eyes.

How do these lenses work? The cornea (the clear dome that sits over the iris) is made of a collagen-like material that is very elastic. Special contact lenses mold it overnight in a precise way based on measurements of the cornea that are taken before this process begins. The results of this therapy last indefinitely, as long as you wear the reshaping lenses every night (in some cases, every other night).

While there are limits to this process if your vision condition is quite severe, corneal molding (sometimes referred to as orthokeratology or corneal refractive therapy) is a far less invasive procedure that provides similar results to LASIK (and in some cases, better results) without the inherent risks of surgery.

LASIK

LASIK (laser-assisted in situ keratomileusis), also known as laser eye surgery, is a procedure designed to improve eyesight that has caught on with the athlete population over the past ten years. Who wouldn't want to see clearly without the encumbrances and inconveniences created by eyeglasses or contact lenses? No eyeglass lenses fogging up during competition! No contact lenses shifting out of place when it's time to hit the ball! It sounds great, and to some degree it is. In fact, I would certainly advocate LASIK surgery for athletes between the ages of twenty-two to forty-two who have significant clarity of vision problems and cannot wear contact lenses successfully due to any number of reasons. Dry eyes, visual corrections that are too intricate to correct effectively with eyeglasses or contact lenses, and unusually shaped eyes are some examples of good reasons to consider LASIK. There are, however, caveats that must be addressed.

As people age, they will all generally encounter a condition known as presbyopia, which is simply defined as the loss of ability to focus on near objects. Essentially, the focusing lens of the eye loses elasticity as part of the aging process. LASIK surgery, however, does not resolve this aging problem (in fact, it may exacerbate it). Nor does LASIK guarantee perfect eyesight. In fact, many of my athlete patients experience less clarity of vision after LASIK than they were able to achieve with their previous eyeglasses or contact lenses. Don't forget: LASIK is surgery, and as with any surgery, there is always risk of failure (although the failure rate is relatively small and has improved over the years).

Too often, LASIK is chosen by an athlete simply out of laziness. In this fast-moving world, people have no time for anything inconvenient, and caring for contact lenses is just one of the possible time-consuming obstacles they'd love to avoid. But there are potential ongoing issues following LASIK surgery, including dry eyes (don't forget that the cornea has been cut and therefore compromised by this procedure), halos around lights that do not always improve with healing, glare, and light sensitivity. Granted, these symptoms may improve with time, but that's not always the case.

Of course, even after LASIK surgery, risk of permanent injury to the globe of the eye remains a major concern in many contact sports. On the other hand, a track and field enthusiast might love the freedom from eyeglasses or contacts in competition.

CONCLUSION

If your ultimate goal is to be the best athlete you can be, then I implore you not to forget about the basics. Your eyes must be as healthy as possible. Don't assume they are. Be conscientious and visit your eyecare provider on an annual basis. Be proactive when it comes to eye health. The operative word is prevention. You need to be visually fit to be physically fit. Before you can proceed to implement the training benefits of this book, get your eyes checked.

There is a general misconception that athletes have great eyesight and healthy eyes. The reality is that no matter how old you are or how physically demanding your sport may be, there is always a chance that eye problems exist and may create risks not only on the playing field but also in day-to-day life. Many people are completely unaware of eyesight deficits. Even if one eye sees well, the other eye may not. Too frequently people are unaware that they are not seeing the world as they were meant to see it. In particular, athletes are the biggest culprits when it comes to overlooking potential eye problems. The thought of eye problems is typically the farthest thing from an elite athlete's mind. But even if an eye problem is minimal, seeing with pinpoint vision could mean the difference between a .300 batting average and a .350 batting average.

To paraphrase the great Muhammed Ali, "Float like a butterfly, sting like a bee. Your hands can't hit what your eyes can't see!" In other words, if you hope to play well, it helps to see well. I realize that some great athletes have excelled without the benefit of perfect vision, but I contend that by maximizing visual performance you can achieve athletic excellence. This idea holds true at any age, from child athletes to pros.

3.

Preventing Eye Conditions and Injuries

Perhaps the highest priority before embarking on a high performance vision program is to visit an eyecare professional who will carefully assess your eye health. Athletes of all ages are at risk of injury and disease that can impact their eyes. The first step is prevention, but sometimes things go wrong no matter how cautious you are. Different sports hold different risk factors. If you play your sport outdoors, environmental factors like wind, dust, and temperature could lead to potential eye problems or injuries.

EYE CONDITIONS

Today's advanced computer technology can produce detailed information about all the critical structures of a patient's eyes. For example, the retina, the back inside layer of the eye, cannot be seen clearly without the help of technology. Obviously, some sports are more likely than others to cause trauma to the retina. It is essential that the retina of an athlete who participates in contact sports such as ice hockey, football, and boxing be carefully examined. It should not be assumed, however, that retinal issues are limited only to these activities.

A baseline analysis of retinal health should be established before an athlete starts a sports season. The status of the retina should then be reexamined annually. Moreover, the retina is not the only part of the eye that can be damaged. Here are some typical eye problems and their potential remedies. This information can help you avoid the ocular obstacles that may be standing between you and a successful day on the playing field.

Blepharitis

Allergies can wreak havoc on your eyes. Blepharitis is a condition that causes eyelids to become red, itchy, and scaly. Skin allergies can provoke this problem. A bacterial infection of the eyelids may also be the culprit. Most recently, a small eyelash mite called *Demodex* has been linked to many cases of blepharitis.

Following proper eyelid hygiene and scrubbing the lids with products such as Cliradex may help resolve this condition.

Cataract

A cataract, by definition, is an opaque discoloration of the lens of the eye. Perhaps more than most people, athletes are at particular risk of cataract, but why is this so? Science tells us that excessive exposure to harmful violet and ultraviolet light rays can cause discoloration of the lens of the eye. If your sport is played outdoors, over a lifetime you are at greater risk of developing a cataract. One particular target group that exemplifies this risk is senior golfers.

So, what can you do to reduce your risk of cataract? If possible when playing your sport, wear UV-shielding sunglasses that offer full UV protection. If your game precludes the use of sunglasses, you should be aware that some contact lenses are designed to filter out significant amounts of UV rays. Ask your eyecare professional to consider fitting you with these contact lenses. At the very least, a hat with a brim may help to some degree.

Conjunctivitis (Pink Eye)

We've all heard of it, and, yes, we can all get it. Some may not know the medical designation conjunctivitis, but most have heard the term "pink eye." So, what is it? It's an inflammation of the membrane that covers the eyeball and inside of the eyelids. Conjunctivitis typically makes your eyes look red. They may also tear profusely. How can you avoid it? For one, don't rub your eyes! Secondly, keep dirty fingers, towels, and any foreign objects away from your eyes. Think of sports such as baseball, for example. The game is played on dirt and the players often rub that dirt onto their hands when batting. Athletes also share locker rooms, where bacteria and viruses can easily spread. If there is itchiness involved, however, allergies may be the culprit.

To summarize, pink eye can come from bacteria, a virus, or allergies. Therefore, it must be treated appropriately. When pink eye is caused by bacteria, the problem is usually treated with an antibiotic eye drop. If allergies are behind the condition, an anti-itch drop may also be beneficial and provide relief from symptoms. Viral conjunctivitis is typically the most difficult type of pink eye to treat. It can last for quite a long time, sometimes up to a month. It is also highly contagious. Athletes who have viral conjunctivitis must avoid any hand contact, touching of their eyes, or situations in which towels are shared.

Dry Eye

Dry eye is a condition that has reached epidemic proportions in the United States. The outer layer of the human eye needs sufficient lubrication to ensure clarity of vision and eye comfort. An athlete cannot afford to experience blurred, hazy vision at the moment of truth, when she is at a critical moment and must perform successfully in her sport. Dry eye problems are definitely more prevalent with age, but athletes of all ages risk dealing with this condition. When it comes to dry eye, sports that particularly come to mind are outdoor activities such as baseball, golf, tennis, auto racing, and soccer—although indoor sports such as ice hockey and basketball can also be a concern due to the drying effect that air conditioning has on the surface of the eyes. The tear layer of the surface of the eye is constantly at risk of dryness as a result of diet, genetics, lack of a full blink reflex, and environmental issues such as wind, dust, and pollution.

Symptoms of dry eye may include excessive blinking, a gritty feeling in the eyes, itching, redness, and, in some cases, haziness in the field of vision. Many over-the-counter artificial tears offer varying degrees of viscosity (lubrication) and are available in pharmacies. Additionally, omega-3 supplements may be effective when taken daily to ward off problems associated with dry eye.

Pinguecula and Pterygium

There are two eye conditions that occur more frequently in the athlete population than in the general population. Their medical names are pinguecula and pterygium. Simply put, a pinguecula is a growth that appears on the clear membrane, or conjunctiva, which sits over the white part of the eye known as the sclera. It is typically caused by excessive exposure to sunlight, wind, or dust. According to my many years of medical practice, the athletes that display this problem with the greatest frequency are tennis players, golfers, skiers, and, in general, athletes who compete under constant bombardment from ultraviolet or blue-violet light. For example, I would often see pinguecula growths on the eyes of numerous baseball players who grew up in South America, Mexico, or on islands in the Caribbean. I would also observe this condition more frequently in blue-eyed, fair-skinned individuals.

The difference between a pinguecula and a pterygium is the extent of growth of the mass on the eye. A pinguecula is typically limited to the white of the eye, whereas a pterygium starts to encroach on the cornea in the zone where the colored part of the eye, or iris, is situated. The greatest risk associated with a pterygium is that it can grow to a position that blocks the pupil.

Wearing high-quality full-spectrum sunglasses is a good way to protect against these growths. If need be, these problems may be removed with a treatment involving a laser device.

SPORT-RELATED EYE INJURIES

The number of eye injuries that occur during the heat of athletic competition continues to be of concern as more and more people become active in sports and recreation. The following are a few of the most prevalent injuries that can damage the eyes and, in some cases, lead to loss of sight.

Corneal Abrasion

The cornea is the clear dome that covers the iris (the colored part of the eye). Its transparency allows usable light to reach the back of the eyes and provide the images we see. A scratch or gouge to the cornea can cause serious pain, tearing, and blurred vision, which will impair your ability to participate in sports. Often a corneal abrasion may occur as a result of a foreign particle becoming imbedded in the cornea. Any foreign body in the cornea or abrasion to the cornea demands that you see a doctor as soon as possible. Typically, a topical antibiotic will be used as treatment. A cycloplegia drop may also be used to prevent the pupil from pulsating and creating pain. If warranted due to significant discomfort while blinking, an FDA-approved overnight soft contact lens may be used as a bandage lens until the abrasion begins to heal. In rare cases, an over-the-counter pain killer such as ibuprofen may be needed. After a corneal abrasion heals, it is important to be aware that the previously damaged area of your eye can become reinjured. This is referred to as "recurrent corneal erosion." Another visit to your doctor may be necessary to deal with this complication.

Detached Retina

Athletes, especially those who play contact sports, are at greater risk than most of tearing the back inner wall of the eye. When this happens, it is referred to as a detached retina. Often the first sign of a retinal detachment is "lightning flashes" seen somewhere in the field of vision. More extensive tears can result in a partial or total curtain-like shadow in the field of vision. An athlete may not notice this shadow if the other eye is intact. It behooves the athlete to close each eye separately and compare the individual fields of vision. Flashes of light or large floating objects in a person's vision may indicate that the gel-like material in front of the retina (the vitreous humor) has been torn. Although requiring a doctor's care, a detached vitreous is of less concern than a detached retina. Often, the best treatment with this condition is taking a break from strenuous exercise for a few weeks and monitoring the symptoms. Obviously, any increase in symptoms should be reevaluated by your doctor. Anyone with a suspected detached retina should see a trained retinal surgeon immediately to confirm the extent of the problem. The severity of the tear will dictate the course of action to be followed.

Minor tears can be repaired by welding the torn area with a laser. More extensive detachments need to be surgically reattached and monitored over several weeks to months. In some cases, an athlete may be prevented from returning to competition, either temporarily or permanently.

Hyphema

When a significant blow to the eye causes extensive trauma, one possible outcome is blood leaking into the anterior chamber of the globe. This type of injury is known as hyphema. Immediate treatment of this condition calls for immobilization of the eye with an eye shield and restriction of physical activity. A cycloplegia drop may be used to paralyze the pupil and prevent it from dilating or constricting. In addition, a topical corticosteroid may be employed to combat inflammation to the injured components of the eye. If you are recovering from a hyphema, your doctor should monitor you for re-bleeds and increased pressure in the eye (acute glaucoma). Initially, your eye may be dilated to allow a more expansive view of the internal structures of the back wall of your eye.

Lid Laceration

A blow to the eye can result in a laceration, or significant tear to the eyelid. Besides suturing the wound, your doctor will need to rule out any additional ocular damage and check for any possible foreign objects imbedded in the lid wound or anywhere else in your eye.

Orbital Trauma (Blowout Fracture)

Trauma to an eye can also result in significant damage to the bones that surround the globe. These bones are referred to as the ocular orbit, and damage to them is described as a blowout fracture. If this type of major trauma occurs, your doctor will carefully investigate the movement of your eyes in all positions of gaze. It is probable that a CT scan will be ordered to assess the extent of the damage in greater detail. This injury warrants careful monitoring and possibly surgery if it is accompanied by persistent double vision.

Ruptured or Lacerated Globe

A ruptured or lacerated globe is a rather serious condition that needs immediate treatment. The extent of rupture or laceration needs to be assessed and the internal pressure of the eye needs to be measured to determine if there is a sudden drop off in pressure. A metal eye shield needs to be put in place. A standard eye patch should be avoided because it can cause additional pressure on the ocular surface.

Impaired Vision from Concussion or Head Trauma

The buzz word in sports medicine today is "concussion." Everywhere you look, people are expounding on the impact concussions have on athletes. It has become the focus of concern in all sports where trauma occurs. More often than not, the eyes are impacted by

35

the neurological deficits that accompany a blow to the head. The following information details the visual symptoms that can accompany a concussion.

Blurred Vision

Blurred vision following a concussion may occur in the far or near field, or in both.

Convergence Insufficiency

This inability to use the eyes comfortably in the near field may result in a number of symptoms, including headache, eye strain, eye fatigue, and even double vision during near-field activities.

Double Vision (Diplopia)

If an athlete reports any degree of double vision, whether constant or intermittent, a careful evaluation of the eyes by a trained professional is advised.

Tracking Deficits

Deficiencies in eye movement are quite common following a concussion or another form of mild traumatic brain injury. Invariably, this condition will significantly impact an athlete's playing performance in an adverse way.

Focusing at Near

Whereas young athletes with no history of concussion generally have no difficulty zeroing in on an object as it draws near, post-concussion athletes of all ages may suffer from constantly blurred vision, or may have visual clarity that comes and goes during near-field activities.

Light Sensitivity (Photophobia)

A significant number of athletes report light sensitivity a major symptom after experiencing a concussion. Interestingly, this condition mimics a similar symptom reported by migraine sufferers.

Reduced Cognitive Ability in Visual Tasks

Visual perceptual deficits, including visual memory, visual sequencing of letters or numbers, and visual concentration, may be caused by concussion and have dramatic effects on athletic success.

Reduced Visual Reaction Time

Visual processing speed may slow down after head trauma. This reduced speed of reaction can impair an athlete's ability to read the field of play, judge the speed of a moving ball or puck, or recognize the speed of movement of other players on the field.

Preventing Concussion

Prevention of concussion starts with improved protective headgear designs. Modern polymers have allowed equipment manufacturers

First Aid Kit for Ocular Emergencies

Athletic trainers have become prevalent at all levels of competition, from middle school to the pros. These dedicated professionals are well versed in treating athletic injuries of all kinds. Many trainers, however, will admit to a limited understanding of eye-related first aid. With demand growing for on-field first aid for potential eye injuries, it is important to know which items should be required in a kit. The following materials should suffice for anyone wishing to address ocular trauma.

- Ice pack
- Mirror
- Spare contact lenses
- Saline
- Irrigating solution
- Ocular anesthetic
- Penlights (white and blue lights)
- Medical tape
- Sani-wipes
- Fluorescein strips
- DMV contact lens remover
- Q-tips
- Fox aluminum eye shield
- Nearpoint vision card
- Cotton eye pads

to create helmets that cushion significant blows to the head. Perhaps as important is a mandatory requirement that headgear be worn by athletes under all playing conditions. Unfortunately, treatment of head trauma, or CTE (chronic traumatic encephalopathy), is limited to early detection of brain damage and the implementation of various psychotropic drugs to reduce accompanying symptoms.

PROTECTIVE EYEWEAR

I was recently asked to testify as an expert witness in a lawsuit in which a youngster taking part in a high school floor hockey game shot a puck after the game had ended. The puck struck another player in the eye, detaching his retina and damaging the globe. Although this was an unintentional accident (the youngster who shot the puck wasn't thinking and was letting out some frustration on the puck), blame was directed not only at the frustrated player but also at the high school. It was argued (and I agreed) that the school was negligent because it should have made protective eyewear (in this case, a face shield) mandatory for all students participating in this or any other school sport.

The lesson to be learned here is that protective eyewear should be an accepted part of equipment for just about every youth sport. Obviously, this eyewear needs to be tougher than standard eyeglasses worn on a daily basis. Additionally, specific sports need to use specific eye protection.

Basketball

The goggles worn in basketball should allow for a wide field of view, and be durable, fog-resistant, and anchor securely to the head with a headband. There are a number of good choices on the market, but I prefer the Victory line of goggles by Hilco. It has a distinctive bubble design and provides a 180-degree peripheral field of vision. It meets impact standards set by the American Society for Testing and Materials (ASTM) and is made of polycarbonate. It is also well ventilated with its flow-through side vents.

Racquet Sports

Tough, lightweight eye protection is essential for tennis and racquetball. A scratch-resistant polycarbonate lens is advised. One beneficial technology in tennis is the Competivision lens by Bolle. Its unusual blue-green filter eliminates transmission of all colors of the spectrum except optic yellow. As a result, many players who wear these lenses claim that the tennis ball seems to pop out of the background. As for racquet sports such as squash or racquetball, I would recommend the Action Eyes frame by Black Knight USA. Its shape more closely resembles a standard eyeglass frame, but it has a reinforced rubberized bridge, seven barrel hinges, and a retainer headband. Its large lens design provides a wide peripheral view and resists fogging better than many wraparound designs.

Skiing

Several ski masks may be adapted for inclusion of prescription lens inserts. Bolle's Xeno and Helix ski masks, for example, have an antifog double vented lens and are available in several lens tints. The Helix is especially suited to the smaller faces of children.

Swimming and Water Sports

Many manufacturers offer prescription swim goggles. It is even possible to get swimming caps with built-in prescription lenses. Some examples include Ducal Trading's Child's Rxable Swim Goggles, Aqua Specs AQ-1 by Liberty, Speedo Jr. Pro by Opti-Sport, and the Sable WaterOptics RS 922. Many diving and snorkeling masks are available from these manufacturers as well. In fact, Scuba Spec, Inc. makes a prescription lens insert with a unique anchor bar that attaches to the faceplate of the mask. This company also offers the Snorkel Spec #137 EBP insert, which adheres to the faceplate by means of a suction cup.

Hockey and Football

Both these sports warrant critical eye protection. As stated earlier, eye-protective gear should be mandatory in youth sports, and certainly in hockey and football. While football face shields serve to ward off eye injuries, they may also give quarterbacks the advantage of preventing the defense from determining the direction in which the ball will be thrown before the pass is made.

Additional Eye Protection

Protective eyewear may be found for a variety of other sports as well. For example, there are goggles designed for bicycling, lacrosse, field hockey, and paintball. If you are active recreationally, it is important to familiarize yourself with the vast array of protective eyewear options that exist today.

In addition, it's never too early to shield your eyes from the sun's harmful rays. Even as children, it is important to block out ultraviolet, violet, and blue light from the eyes. The good thing is that most children love choosing and wearing their own sunglasses, so getting them to protect their eyes should not be difficult. As previously mentioned, ultraviolet light has been linked to cataract formation in later life. Blue and violet wavelengths penetrate the globe to the retina, where they can damage the macula or produce melanomas. Sadly, my practice once diagnosed a fifteen-year-old field hockey player with melanoma. Perhaps this horrible tumor could have been avoided with the right eye protection.

Several manufacturers, including Oakley, Bolle, Maui Jim, and Vedalo, produce outstanding lens coatings to shield eyes from the sun. Dr. Jim Gallas of Photoprotective Technologies has even developed melanin sunglass lenses. They are purported to filter out all ultraviolet, violet, and blue wavelengths for maximum eye protection. They may be polarized, provide excellent contrast, and do not distort natural colors.

NUTRITIONAL SUPPLEMENTS

Emerging research suggests that nutrition plays a critical role in an athlete's visual performance. The family of nutrients known as carotenoids seems to hold promise for improving eye health. One of them, dietary zeaxanthin, a nutrient scarce in the average American diet, is clinically proven to improve visual function in athletes and young healthy adults at higher doses. Combined with lutein, dietary zeaxanthin accumulates towards the back of the eye to form macular pigment. Macular pigment functions as a set of internal polarized sunglasses to enhance and protect the quality of your vision. Research has demonstrated that over a three-month time period, supplementation with dietary zeaxanthin improves contrast sensitivity, glare recovery, color saturation, and light sensitivity, among other important visual traits. New clinical research has demonstrated the positive role of dietary zeaxanthin on neural efficiency, as this nutrient is also absorbed into the brain. A double-blind, placebo-controlled study conducted by the University of Georgia showed that supplementation with 26 mg of dietary zeaxanthin over a four-month time frame can improve visual-processing speed, or the speed at which eyes process information, by 12 percent and reaction time by 10 percent.

Based on this emerging zeaxanthin research, a St. Louis-based company, Zeavision, has created EyePromise vizual EDGE PRO, a dietary supplement featuring 26 mg of dietary zeaxanthin. This supplement has been certified by the National Science Foundation (NSF) to ensure athletes that it is absolutely free of the over 180 banned substances on the MLB, NCAA, NFL, and WADA lists of banned substances.

CONCLUSION

There are numerous eye health issues that can interfere with your playing performance. I've touched upon only a few prevalent examples. Athletes must be cognizant of the fact that the possibility of eye injury accompanies almost any form of sporting competition. Furthermore, an ounce of prevention is worth a pound of cure. It behooves athletes, coaches, trainers, and parents to recognize the need for proper protective eyewear, which can prevent serious consequences on the playing field. The message is simply this: Your eyes must stay healthy in order for you to play at your optimum level.

4.

Measuring Your Visual Skills

Good vision is important not just in athletics but in life in general. While most people consider 20/20 vision the ideal, it is not nearly sufficient to put you on the road to becoming a high-level athlete. A trained eyecare professional that is proficient in evaluating and training the high performance vision skills of athletes can administer certain tests to determine how you may achieve your highest possible power of sight. These sport-specific examinations are often undertaken during a follow-up visit, after a comprehensive standard eye examination has been completed. This sports-related battery of tests can take anywhere from ninety minutes to two hours to complete. Many of these procedures are conducted on every type of athlete. In addition, tests designed for specific sports allow doctors to pinpoint abilities that are most relevant to a particular sport. Although challenging, these examinations can reveal significant visual strengths and weaknesses. The work-up is enjoyable to do, and may even stimulate your competitive juices as an athlete. This chapter will describe a number of visually driven skills, with a focus on how these particular skills are assessed and measured.

Although I highly recommend you complete a professional vision evaluation before embarking on a professionally assisted high performance vision training program, many of the exercises appearing throughout this book may be executed on your own if you have the proper equipment. The difference between performing them on your own and enlisting the aid of a trainer is structure. A structured program that follows a sequence of skill development will more likely provide a higher level of improvement than a self-guided approach.

ALIGNMENT

Your eyes guide you to a precise point in space and help you to make accurate judgments. They are the mechanism that allows you to estimate the distance between the ball and its target. Perfect alignment allows for a precise match between where you perceive objects to be and where they actually are. If your eyes are aiming closer or farther than you think, it's no wonder that you consistently come up short or long when putting for that birdie, when needing to make a critical foul shot, or when trying to hit the ball to right field. A simple way to assess your eye muscle alignment is to set your sights on a small object (perhaps a doorknob, for example) that is located at a distance greater than eight feet away. Rapidly alternate covering each eye and note whether this object shifts dramatically from side to side or up and down. A significant displacement of the target could indicate a flaw in eye-muscle alignment. A practitioner of high performance vision training can measure your alignment in free space using a Maddox Rod (see Figure 4.1) and Phoria Card (see Figure 4.2). The eyes are evaluated for alignment with the following potential outcomes:

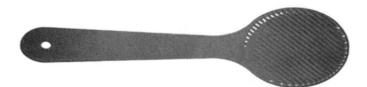

Figure 4.1. Maddox Rod

A translucent red paddle with parallel lines on its surface, the Maddox Rod measures the alignment of the two eyes working as a team.

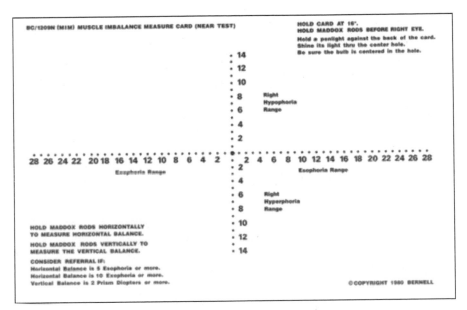

Figure 4.2. Phoria Card

When used in conjunction with a Maddox Rod and a penlight illuminated at the hole in the center of the card, this tool measures eye alignment in units called prism diopters.

Esophoria. Both eyes align closer than the object being viewed.

Exophoria. Both eyes align further away than the object being viewed.

Hyperphoria. One eye is aimed higher than the other.

Hypophoria. One eye is aimed lower than the other.

Orthophoria. Both eyes are aligned in space exactly on the target of regard.

The suffix "tropia" is used to define the extreme versions of these eye conditions. In a tropia, one or both eyes are fixed in a particular locked position and will not move from that position.

ANTICIPATION TIMING

The amount of time it takes to determine where and when an object and an athletic movement will coincide is referred to as anticipation timing. In other words, what is your ability to visually time a moving object and respond motorically? An example would be a pole vaulter's ability to judge where and when to plant the pole for a jump. This timing skill is typically measured in milliseconds.

The Bassin Anticipation Timer (B.A.T.) by Lafayette Instrument Company (see Figure 4.3) evaluates anticipation timing. This instrument consists of a series of three-foot attachable tracks that may be set up on tripods. Each track has a sequence of equally spaced red lights that may be activated by remote control. These lights may be triggered to travel in preset sequences that can be programmed at any speed. The athlete is asked to hit a trigger button or break the plane of a motion sensor in anticipation of the final light on the track illuminating. The remote control will record in milliseconds whether the athlete's timing is early or late. The B.A.T. is an excellent way to evaluate such timing skills as hitting a baseball or tennis ball, shooting skeet, or stopping a hockey puck from reaching the goal.

COLOR VISION

Most people have been genetically blessed with the ability to recognize the various colors of the spectrum rapidly and accurately. Having this talent is imperative in many sports, especially when it comes to seeing an object such as a ball or puck against a particular background. This ability also plays a major role in allowing an athlete to discriminate between the uniform of teammates and that of the opposing team. Statistically, almost 10 percent of all males struggle to identify colors like red, orange, green, blue, magenta, and yellow. The percentage of females with color vision deficits is much smaller (approximating half of 1 percent). The degree of color vision loss varies by individual. The typical red-green defect in its extreme form is called protanopia (reds, oranges, blues, and magenta) or deuteranopia (greens and yellows). The milder versions of each are termed protanomaly and deuteranomaly, respectively. Many of you have heard of the rods and cones on the inside back wall of the eye. These are the receptors that allow us a sense of sight. Rods deal with

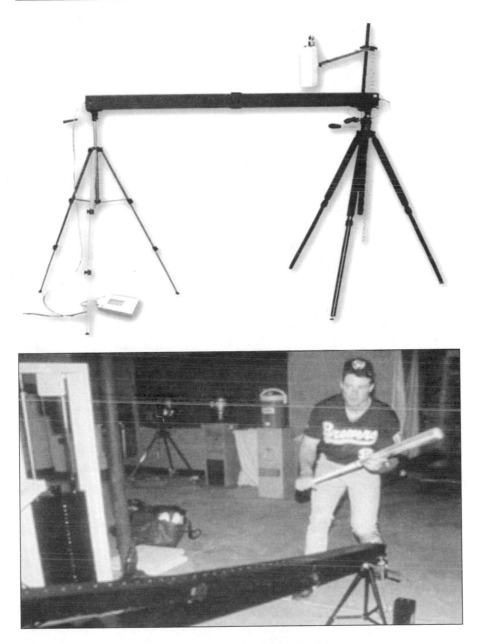

Figure 4.3. Bassin Anticipation Timer

This device has a series of electronically triggered LED lights, which simulate the movement of an object towards or away from the test subject. In the example above, the batter must swing the bat when the lights reach a certain point.

night vision predominantly, while cones are critical for crisp, clear vision during daylight hours. In addition, it is the cones that provide accurate color vision.

Athletes have asked me whether there are people who see no colors except black and white. This condition is extremely rare, but it does exist. These individuals are called monochromats. Specially tinted colored glasses or contact lenses may, in some instances, help improve color discrimination problems. The X-Chrom lens is a popular contact lens that has been used to provide greater appreciation of colors. It is available in both gas-permeable (firm) lens material and the more popular soft lens polymer.

It should be noted that some diseases and medications have adverse effects on color discrimination. A high performance vision specialist can evaluate an athlete's color appreciation skill with tests like the Ishihara Color Test and the Pseudoisochromatic Plate (PIP) Color Vision Test. The doctor can also assess the degree of skill an athlete demonstrates in his ability to distinguish between different intensities of colors (known as hue discrimination) by employing the Farnsworth-Munsell D-15 test. In this examination, the patient is asked to match different shades of colors on discs compared side by side.

Defects in color vision can make it difficult for a quarterback to spot a receiver, to distinguish a team member from a competitor, and to follow accurately an object in motion. Color vision deficits also explain why some golfers have difficulty seeing an orange or yellow ball on the fairway. I am reminded of a situation that I participated in with former NFL quarterback, Vinny Testaverde. When Vinny was starting for the Tampa Bay Buccaneers, I had the opportunity to evaluate the visual performance skills of the entire roster of players. It had been known that Vinny suffered from color blindness, so I recommended that he be fitted for an X-Chrom lens, which would be worn on his non-dominant eye. The week following the fitting, the Bucs were scheduled to play an away game against the Green Bay Packers. The Packers' coaching staff had been made aware of Vinny's color vision issues, so they chose to wear their away uniforms (which are green and gold) even though they were the home team. The Bucs wore their orange uniforms. The Packers coaches were hoping to confuse Testaverde when he needed to find a receiver in an instant. Remember, people who are color-vision deficient have a hard time distinguishing between colors such as red, green, and orange. Unbeknownst to the Packers, Vinny was wearing his new X-Chrom lens and proceeded to have an incredibly successful passing day. Tampa Bay won the game. *Sports Illustrated* even picked up the story, revealing the details of this "chess game" in their next issue.

CONTRAST SENSITIVITY

This is the ability of an athlete to discern fine detail differences (for example, seeing black on white to appreciate changes in contours) in his field of view. As the brightness and color of the background approach that of the object being tracked, contrast between this object and the background diminishes. Having outstanding visual acuity does not necessarily equate with skill in contrast interpretation. Deficits in this ability could make it difficult for an athlete to "pick up" and "stay on" any object that needs to be followed. The athlete would have a tendency to be slow to notice an object and would, therefore, lose balls, pucks, people, etc. Those who are gifted with outstanding contrast sensitivity are purported to see the stitches and rotation of a pitched baseball, the contours of a ski slope, and the location of an orange clay pigeon against a blue sky better than their competitors, to name but a few examples.

Equipment such as the CSV-1000 by VectorVision (see Figure 4.4) will allow your doctor to quantify your contrast sensitivity. Using this device, you will be asked to select the circles that contain the same vertically oriented fine lines, or sine-wave gratings, as the example found at the beginning of each row. The test includes four rows with eight comparisons displayed in each row. A numerical score can be calculated and compared to norms that have been established for this high performance vision category.

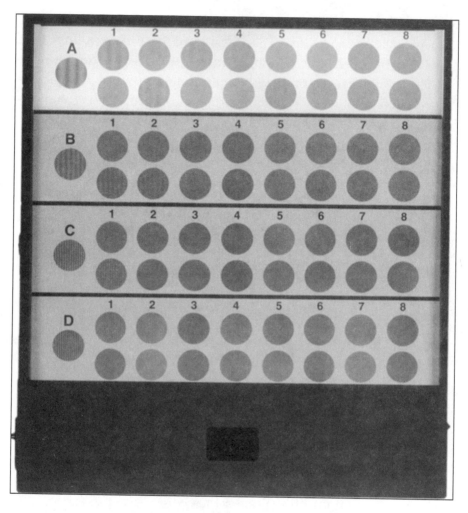

Figure 4.4. CSV-1000 by VectorVision

Illuminated box with increasingly difficult contrast gradient targets vertically displayed to measure the test subject's ability to appreciate fine detail.

DEPTH PERCEPTION

Depth perception, or stereopsis, is the ability to interpret the combined images from both eyes to judge distances, speeds, and spatial relationships rapidly and precisely. It is intimately related to accurate eye movement and the flexibility of both eyes as they work together as a team. For example, in the game of tennis, experts rate outstanding depth perception as the most important visual attribute to possess, even above court speed and eye-hand coordination. This skill may be diminished, however, by extended near work prior to a tennis match. Appropriately, a number of studies have shown that students, computer programmers, and workers whose jobs require extensive close work play much poorer tennis after work than on weekends.

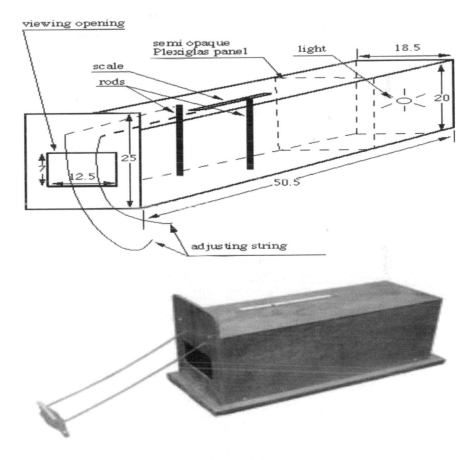

Figure 4.5. Howard-Dolman Apparatus

This device measures depth perception by requiring the test subject to align two posts so that they are positioned side by side within the viewing box.

Deficits in depth perception can cause athletes to misjudge where they are in relation to other objects on the field of play. It can also result in an athlete misinterpreting where objects are in relation to other objects. The most realistic place to evaluate your depth perception is by simulating playing conditions. The Howard-Dolman Apparatus (see Figure 4.5) is a simple but effective instrument to test depth perception. This equipment is nothing more than two strings attached to separate posts that can be pulled within an enclosed box. During the examination, the test subject's task is to align one of the two posts side by side with the other while viewing them at eight feet or beyond. Scoring is accomplished by measuring the discrepancy between the two posts at the completion of the task (in millimeters). If an athlete consistently misjudges the outcome by choosing a position at which the moveable post is farther away than the fixed post or vice versa, a reason for poor spatial judgment may be determined.

THE DOMINANT EYE

The dominant eye is also referred to as the preferred eye or the aiming eye. It is the eye with which you align objects in the process of seeing with both eyes. The fact is that both eyes are never fixed on the object of regard at the same time. One eye leads and the other follows. If both eyes were able to focus at exactly the same point in space at the same time, then we would not be able to see the world in three dimensions, and we would certainly have very poor depth perception.

There is a general misconception that the dominant eye is the eye that sees most clearly of the two eyes. In reality, because eye dominance is predetermined genetically, visual development throughout a lifetime is unrelated to eye dominance. In fact, the dominant eye, in some cases, may have poorer vision than the non-dominant eye. It is also untrue that eye dominance must coincide with the preferred hand or foot. Statistically, neurologists have found that approximately 80 percent of right-handed people are right-eyed as well. This means the remaining 20 percent are of cross or mixed dominance. Among southpaws, the results are even more astounding. About 60 percent of all lefties are left-eyed, but a significant 40 percent are right-eye dominant. This may explain the preponderance of ambidextrous lefties. It should also be pointed out that eye dominance cannot truly be changed, nor should it. Studies have shown that forcing this action can lead to other issues, including stuttering and confusion, in adulthood. Although rare, some people demonstrate a true equal dominance in which aim can switch between one eye and the other.

To determine your dominant eye, fixate on a small object at a distance (greater than eight feet away). This can be a doorknob or any object at eye level. Extend both arms fully in front of you while forming a small triangular opening between your two hands. Set

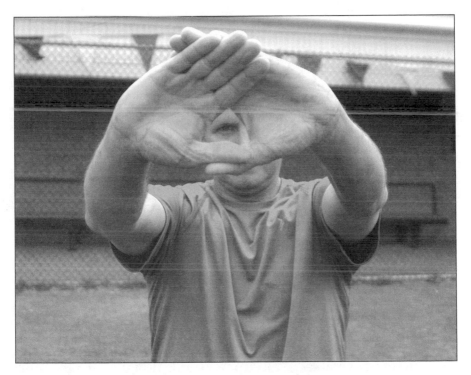

Figure 4.6. Dominant Eye Test
Proper positioning of the hands to determine which eye is dominant.

the sight of your object of regard through the triangle and then shut one eye at a time. Observe which eye's line of vision remains on the doorknob. This is your dominant eye. (See Figure 4.6.)

In 1980, I had the unique opportunity to study the relationship of eye dominance to hand dominance in 270 major league baseball players from seven teams. With reference to the relationship between the dominant or preferred (aiming) eye and the dominant hand, the results were astonishing. Exactly 50 percent of the entire test population was found to have cross-dominance (left-handed and right-eyed, or right-handed and left-eyed). Interestingly, teams with a high percentage of cross-dominant players had better batting averages than those without. The Kansas City Royals, who led the major leagues in batting average in 1980, had a remarkable 70 percent rate of cross-dominance. (The general populace approximates 20 percent at most.)

EYE-HAND-FOOT COORDINATION

I have intentionally used the term "eye-hand coordination" and not "hand-eye coordination" as it is sometimes inaccurately stated. After all, the eyes always lead the body (hands and feet). To make an analogy, each human is a very sophisticated closed-loop computer system. The sensory system, approximately 80 percent of which is controlled by the eyes, is the input component. Data is fed to the brain through an intricate nerve network. The brain is the processor. Finally, the body (or motor system) is the final output for this amazing closed-loop system known as human being.

Eye-hand-foot coordination involves the integration of the eyes and the hands and feet as a unit. The eyes must lead and guide the motor (movement) system of the body. Deficits in this ability can affect all facets of athletics. There is a multitude of equipment that has been developed to evaluate and train this critical skill for athletic success. Several large electronic boards designed for this purpose are available. They have such varied names as the SVT, the Action Coach, the Sanet Vision Integrator, the Visual Motor

Enhancement System (VMET), the Wayne Saccadic Fixator, DynaVision, and the Nike SPARQ System. They all concentrate on assessing and improving visual-motor performance by asking the athlete being tested to touch randomly illuminated lights within a predetermined time limit. Devices such as the Reaction Plus and MOART (Multi Operational Apparatus for Reaction Time) also incorporate eye-to-foot reaction tests.

EYE-MOVEMENT SKILL

Eye-movement skill (eye tracking, ocular motility) is defined as the ability of the two eyes to perform together as the athlete looks from place to place or follows a moving target. This skill is used whether an athlete or target is in motion or stationary. Eye tracking is critical in most sports. It has been demonstrated that an athlete will excel in a chosen sport when head movement is minimized and eye-tracking movement is maximized. Deficits in eye-movement skill can affect judgment of spatial orientation, spatial relationships, and depth perception, as well as the need for immediate clear vision of all objects in the field of view.

Three types of eye movement influence the accuracy of how a person sees. The first is saccadic eye movement, which is defined as the speed and accuracy with which you look from one object to another. Also known as saccades, these movements are essentially a series of jumps in fixation. The more efficient these eye shifts are, the quicker you pick up needed information when looking from point A to point B. The Developmental Eye Movement (D.E.M.) test measures these saccadic eye shifts.

The second is pursuit, which is the smooth following movement your eyes require to stay focused on a moving object. Try balancing a book on your head while attempting to follow the beam of a flashlight projected onto a wall as it smoothly moves left to right, up and down, and diagonally and circularly. Now, with your own flashlight, attempt to keep your beam superimposed on the first beam in motion. It is not easy.

Finally, Z-axis tracking refers to the eye-tracking movement required to follow a moving object coming at you or moving away from you. This near-far and far-near path is defined as the Z-axis. Watching a tennis ball approach your racket, hitting a baseball, or tracking a clay pigeon as it leaves the trap and travels away from you are all examples of Z-axis paths.

EYE TEAMING (FUSION)

Eye teaming is defined as the ability to fuse the two images from the eyes into one image accurately and rapidly, with the eyes working

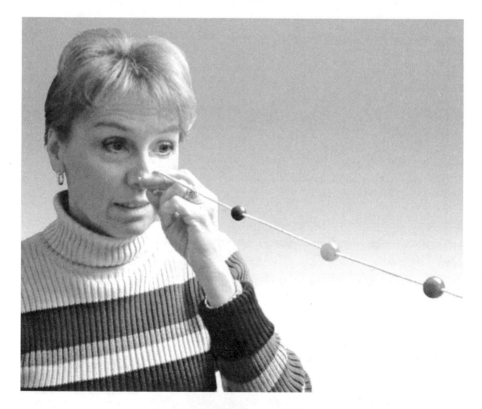

Figure 4.7. Brock String Technique

This tool is simply a string with three beads attached. These beads may be moved along the string to assess eye alignment and teaming.

as a team to maintain this "oneness" in all areas of gaze. Obviously, the better your two eyes can fuse together two images into one image, the greater your depth perception, accuracy in judging distance, and overall quality of vision. Try hitting a golf ball with one eye closed. It can be done, but it's far from easy. This is not to say, however, that we humans cannot be remarkably adaptable and learn to compensate for poor fusion. I have personally seen one-eyed athletes who have managed to achieve impressive levels of success in their respective sports.

The cover test, the Brock String technique (see Figure 4.7), and the Vis-Flex are all useful methods for evaluating the accuracy of visual aim at various distances and positions of gaze.

EYE-TO-FOOT SPEED AND PATTERNING

Without a doubt, the genetic gift of foot speed is predominantly the result of the right DNA. Nevertheless, there are aspects of foot speed that may be trained. After all, the eyes tell the feet what to do and where to go next. With this in mind, let us analyze the components of foot speed:

Raw foot speed. Here's where your DNA and physical fitness come into play. With devices such as the Quick Board (see Figure 6.10), it is now possible to measure in milliseconds how fast an athlete can run various distances.

Eye-foot patterning. Not only do you want to be as fast on your feet as possible, but you need also think on your feet and execute various running patterns with proficiency.

Eye-foot reaction time. This component of foot quickness assesses and trains how quickly you react visually to get your feet where they need to go. An example in the game of baseball would be a base runner getting a quick first step while attempting to steal a base. Devices such as the Reaction Plus (see Figure 4.8) and the MOART (see Figure 4.9) may be used to assess and improve reaction time.

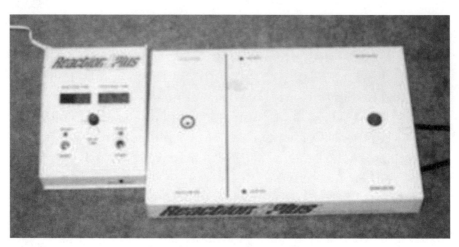

Figure 4.8. Reaction Plus

This electronic device uses lights to measure eye-to-hand reaction time and eye-to-hand response time.

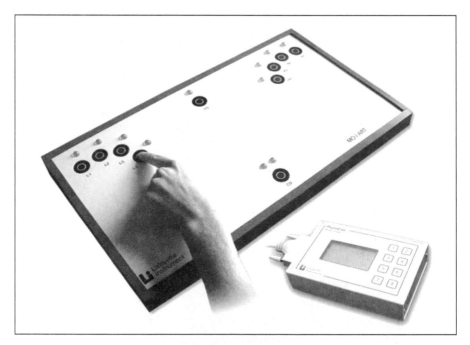

Figure 4.9. MOART

Short for "multi-operational apparatus for reaction time," the MOART is a more sophisticated version of the Reaction Plus, providing a multitude of combinations of lights.

FOCUS FLEXIBILITY

Focus flexibility (or accommodation of the lens of the eye) is the action that allows an individual to change focus from one point in space to another rapidly and without excess effort. Focusing and converging (turning the eyes inward as a team to follow an incoming object) and diverging (turning the eyes outward as a team to follow an outgoing object) are visual skills that work in tandem. Sitting immediately behind the eye's pupil (the opening that allows light to pass through the eye to focus on its back wall or retina) is its crystalline lens. This lens, which is made of an elastic collagen-like material, works very much like the zoom lens of a camera. It allows the eye to shift focus from near to far points and vice versa. The brain sends a message to the nerves and muscles that control this

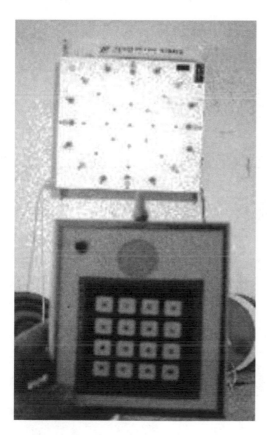

Figure 4.10. Wayne Accommodative Focusing Device

This electronic board has touch-sensitive letters that correspond to letters on a board mounted in the distance.

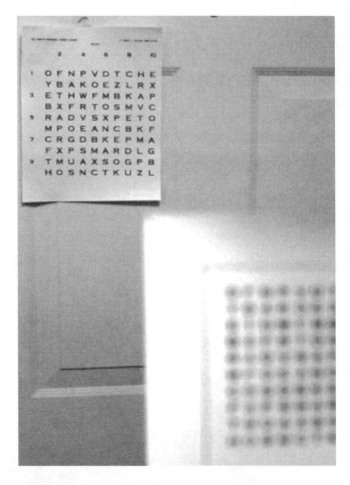

Figure 4.11. Hart Chart

Hart charts have letters randomly displayed in columns. The test subject may use a distance chart and a near chart to enhance focusing ability by shifting from the near chart to the far chart as rapidly as possible.

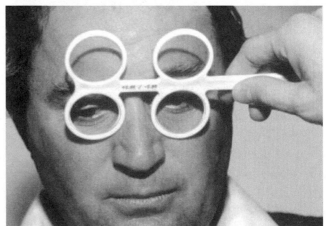

Figure 4.12. Focusing Flippers

This plastic device holds two pairs of lenses, which require the test subject to achieve sharp focus as quickly as possible as they are flipped to change the focusing challenge.

lens, signaling them to flex appropriately to keep images in focus. As humans age, this lens loses elasticity and becomes sluggish in its efforts to get its job done accurately. Deficits in this skill can force an athlete to use excessive effort in the convergence and divergence systems, slowing down the athlete's ability to follow an incoming or outgoing object quickly and accurately. Clarity of all objects could be inconsistent at best and inaccurate at worst.

High performance vision specialists can measure focusing flexibility with devices that include the Wayne Accommodative Focusing Device (see Figure 4.10), Hart Chart (see Figure 4.11), and Focusing Flippers (see Figure 4.12).

EYE-TO-HAND SPEED

I'm sure you have heard someone describe an athlete as having "quick hands." When you think about it, this simply means the athlete has quick eye-to-hand speed. In other words, the athlete's ability to react and respond with his hands to a visual signal is remarkable. Consider the amazing skill required for a batter to accurately hit a ninety-mile-per-hour pitch.

It has often been stated that hitting a fastball in major league baseball is likely the hardest feat to accomplish in athletics. After all, players are voted into the National Baseball Hall of Fame for failing seven out of ten times in their efforts to hit a baseball into fair territory for a base hit. As referenced in an earlier chapter, here are the startling facts: A pitched baseball arrives at home plate in approximately .4 seconds. The batter has .2 seconds to make a visual judgment as to the speed and location of the ball. The batter then has another .2 seconds to make contact with the ball in an effort to get on base. The word "difficult" doesn't begin to explain it.

So, how do high performance vision specialists measure eye-to-hand speed? Two excellent devices that do so are the previously mentioned Reaction Plus and MOART, which are very similar to each other in design and function. They both measure eye-to-hand speed in milliseconds.

Figure 4.13.

HITTING A BASEBALL
So Much to Do, So Little Time (.4 Seconds)

Reprinted from a *New York Times* article, the following is an excellent
graphic portrayal of the components involved in hitting a baseball.

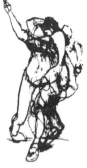

THE RELEASE

1. THE SOFT FOCUS

The batter watches the pitcher's windup with a soft-centered
focus (like a daydream). The eyes are shifted to the pitcher's
release point at the last instance, and the lenses lock onto the
ball. Looking intently at the pitcher too soon will cause the eyes
to get exhausted and lose focus. Some players refer to this
problem as the trance.

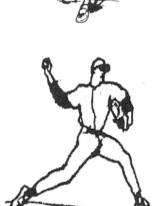

COUNTDOWN TO CONTACT

2. The First .2 Seconds

The batter focuses on the pitcher's release point, while
beginning the backward momentum of the swing. The rotation
of the seams on the ball helps the batter determine the speed
and ultimate location of the pitch. A decision must be made
when and where to swing.

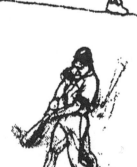

3. The Final .2 Seconds

The final determination of pitch location is made by the hitter,
who in most cases loses sight of the ball as it nears the plate.
As the batter's weight is shifted forward and the hips turn, the
hands throw the barrel of the bat through the path of the ball.

It has often been called the hardest thing to do in sports, and considering that most hitters fail at least 7 out of 10 times, it probably is. Here is a look at some of the mysteries of the batter's box and some of the methods that hitters use to solve them.

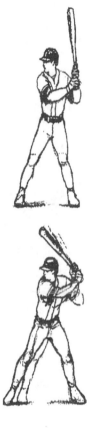

THE SWING

4. Balance and Relaxation

Feet are spread at least shoulder width apart, with weight evenly distributed on both legs. Hands hold the bat softly at the top of the strike zone. All muscles, including the eyes, are relaxed.

5. Stride...

As the pitch is released, a short stride forward is taken and weight is shifted to the back leg. The front shoulder turns inward and the hands move back slowly.

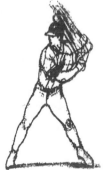

6. ...and Decide

When the speed and location of the pitch is judged, the decision to swing is made. Weight starts forward, hands remain back. Front leg stays slightly bent until contact.

Figure 4.13.   HITTING A BASEBALL (continued)

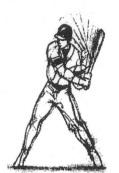

7. Hands and Hips

Hands are thrown downward to the ball, creating the shortest path. The head follows the path of the ball. The back hip and shoulder are thrown toward the ball. Weight continues forward.

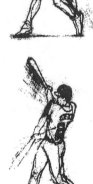

8. Lock and Explode

At contact, the front leg locks, while the back leg and hip explode toward the ball. Front arm is fully extended and the back arm and hand remain behind the bat. Head is pointed toward contact.

9. Extend and Release

The bat continues along the path of the ball to correct the batter's error in timing. The head is released upward, allowing a complete follow-through. Some players release the top hand.

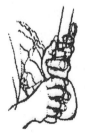

THE LOOSE GRIP

■ It yields a quicker swing because the muscles aren't busy squeezing the bat. The grip becomes firm at contact.

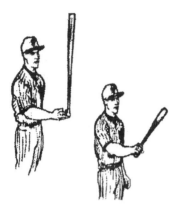

CHOOSING AN ANGLE

■ Some players elect to keep the bat vertical for as long as possible through the swing. The bat appears lighter and the swing is quicker.

■ Although flattening the bat makes it feel heavier, some hitters do so. This gets the bat on the plane of the ball earlier.

SLOW FEET, QUICK HANDS

■ Pitches are thrown at different speeds but look similar when a batter needs to decide to swing. This increases the problem of the batter's timing. A short, slow stride allows the weight to shift backward, while the batter steps forward. This breaks the inertia of the stance without committing the body to the pitch. The stride and the swing are separated, which helps increase timing.

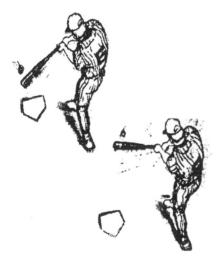

LOCATION, LOCATION

■ Outside pitches, above, need to be hit when the ball is closer to the plate, allowing the swing to stay compact.

■ Inside pitches, below, should be hit well in front of the plate. The swing needs to start in time to get the hips open and the hands through.

GLARE SENSITIVITY AND RECOVERY

Glare sensitivity is a critical component of success in sports. A diminished level of glare sensitivity can be a real hindrance to athletic performance. An athlete's sensitivity to light can impede many aspects of playing ability. Situations in which glare sensitivity can affect the outcome of a game include an outfielder attempting to locate a fly ball in the sun and a tennis player trying to keep an eye on the ball when serving.

Glare recovery refers to the amount of time in milliseconds that it takes the eyes to recover from the powerful impact of glare. It may be measured with a device called a photometer, which measures photosensitivity.

So, what can you do about this potential hazard? Glare-free lenses and antireflective coatings on lenses may help eliminate this problem. Merely tinted sunglasses may also be useful on sun-filled days. There is a group of supplements called carotenoids that help increase pigment in the retina in the light-sensitive zone known as the macula. This increased pigment serves as a protective shield against the sun's harmful rays (ultraviolet A and B, blue light, and infrared light). Carotenoids include the substances lutein, zeaxanthin, and meso-zeaxanthin. They are plentiful in dark green leafy vegetables such as spinach and kale.

NIGHT VISION

Playing a sport outdoors at night under artificial lighting places a different demand on the human eye. Without going into the detailed science of optics, suffice it to say that the retina is composed of information-receiving components called rods and cones. The cones are found in abundance in the macular area (the most critical zone of the retina for providing central vision). The rods are more prevalent in the paramacular area (peripheral to the macula). Although you use both receptors (rods and cones) to see, you depend more on the rods when seeing under nighttime conditions.

Athletes must adapt to darkness when playing at night. It is very important for every athlete to warm up under the lights so that their eyes can acclimate to the extra demand that comes with reduced illumination.

A wonderful instrument for measuring this adaptation skill was developed by the Automobile Association of America (AAA) many years ago. It is called the Night Sight Meter. A simple dial serves as an adjustable resistor, or rheostat, to reduce light gradually while the subject is asked to identify the direction of the opening of a letter "C" as it moves into the line of sight. Norms have been established to rank an individual's ability to accomplish this task.

Vitamin A in the form of beta-carotene (4,000 IU daily) has been shown to enhance one's night vision by increasing the ability of the retina to produce rhodopsin (the biological pigment known also known as visual purple), which is critical to being able to adapt to darkness quickly.

PERIPHERAL FIELD OF VISION

The peripheral field of vision is defined as the full extent of vision extending to 180 degrees while the eyes are focused on a centrally fixed target. The ability of all human beings to appreciate a full field of vision is limited only by anatomical variations such as the protrusion of the nose, cheek bones, and forehead. Various eye diseases and other health conditions may also reduce the peripheral field of vision. It is important to distinguish between the concepts of peripheral vision and peripheral awareness and reaction time. The peripheral field of vision is genetically determined and unchangeable, while peripheral awareness and reaction time may be trained and enhanced. Testing of peripheral vision is typically accomplished through computerized peripheral field-mapping on very sophisticated instruments called field analyzers (see Figure 4.14), which map the field of vision and identify any defects that may exist in that field.

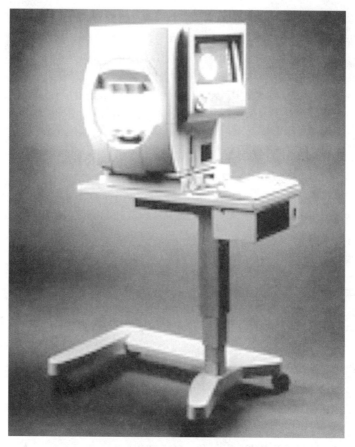

Figure 4.14. Humphrey Field Analyzer

This sophisticated optical instrument electronically maps the field of vision and identifies any defects that may exist in that field.

PERIPHERAL AWARENESS AND REACTION TIME

As mentioned in the previous paragraph, there is a distinction between peripheral vision and peripheral awareness and reaction time. The latter concerns an athlete's ability to pay attention to what is in front of him (central) while being aware of that which is to the side of him (peripheral) without having to move his eyes from the object of regard. In other words, how well do you see out of the corners of your eyes? For example, consider the plight of the marathon runner approaching the finish line. It is almost a necessity to be able to see the competition coming up from the side and behind in order to time your winning acceleration and outrun your opponent.

Deficits in this skill can cause an athlete to lose objects at the sides of where he is looking, and very often to be distracted by objects at the sides of vision. An instrument known as the Peripheral Awareness Trainer by Wayne Engineering (see Figure 4.15) measures the peripheral speed of reaction in milliseconds. It requires the test subject to fixate on a central red light. When the test begins, additional red lights flash randomly from eight peripheral positions of gaze. The goal is to trigger a joystick in the exact direction of the random flashes of light.

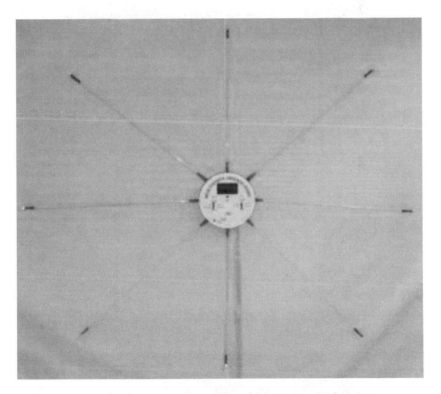

Figure 4.15. Wayne Peripheral Awareness Trainer

This electronic device activates LED lights randomly in the periphery
to test and train peripheral awareness and reaction time.

PROACTION

Just as it pays to be proactive in much of what we do in life, proaction gives an athlete a definitive advantage in sports. A baseball pitcher, for example, may proactively initiate the action of pitching a baseball to a batter. The batter is left with no other option but to react if he wants to succeed. The quicker and more efficiently you can initiate an action, the better your chances are of achieving your goals as an athlete.

You can make this happen because your eyes tell your brain how to activate the nerves and muscles to complete a task at hand, whether it's pitching a baseball, serving a tennis ball, or throwing a forward pass. Many types of equipment can quantify proaction. With all these devices, the subject is asked to identify a sequence of randomly placed lights and then make them change as quickly as possible by tapping them. The more lights the subject accurately taps, the higher the score.

REACTION

Reaction is the time required to perceive and respond to visual stimulation. In other words, the faster you react with precision to a moving object, the better your athletic performance. Also involved in this skill is the ability to utilize auditory information to assist any visual stimulation. For example, take the demands placed on an outfielder to react to the sight and sound of the ball impacting the bat so that he can get a quick first step, run it down, and make the catch. Great reaction time transfers to the playing field. Deficits in this ability may cause some athletes to be slow to respond during sporting activities.

The same equipment that initiates a proaction score may often be programmed to measure reaction scores as well. The difference is that the lights on the device will continue to change at a fixed or random time. The athlete must react quickly enough to these changing lights in order to achieve outstanding results.

REACTION UNDER STRESS

Unfortunately, stress is an expected component of life. In spite of the negative effects of stress on the body, excellence in athletics may be achieved in the face of stressful situations. To some degree, in fact, stress may actually be helpful to athletic performance, stimulating adrenalin flow and allowing your body to kick into fifth gear. It's only when stress is out of control that it becomes a genuine problem. It behooves everyone to learn coping mechanisms to control stress. A few good ways to deal with anxiety include mindful meditation, yoga, visualization, taking a bath, going for a walk in a natural environment, and, thankfully, exercising.

A high performance vision workup will address the impact stress has on your efforts to succeed. Certain pieces of equipment may be used to increase the speed of visual demands and record your attempts to overcome these increased demands on your visual-motor system. One device that evaluates this skill is the Vision Coach. With this equipment, lights are presented randomly while you are asked to touch them in time to react to another light. The stress factor kicks in when these lights begin to accelerate in appearance on the touch board. It is an important ability to master, as failure to react under stress has proven to be one of the major obstacles standing in the way of an athlete's quest for greatness.

REFRACTIVE CONDITION

In today's technology, an automated digital instrument is utilized to evaluate myopia (near-sightedness), hyperopia (far-sightedness), astigmatism, and presbyopia (aging vision). It is critical to correct refractive errors of vision as precisely as possible before any thought is given to improving an athlete's visual-motor skills. After all, you must see at a tremendously high level of proficiency to cope with the demands of most sports.

SPEED OF RECOGNITION

When it comes to sports, speed of recognition refers to an athlete's ability to make quick visual decisions on the playing field. A prime example of this skill is a basketball player attempting to get a shot off or make a pinpoint pass within a fraction of a second while in player traffic.

A tachistoscope is the device of choice to test and train the speed with which an athlete makes visual choices. It can expose images of realistic playing situations at one-hundredth of a second to prompt an accurate response. In the testing mode, numbers may be shown on a screen in various sequences, with the subject asked to report these number sequences correctly. The faster an athlete can make visual decisions about the sports challenge at hand, the more likely he will have a competitive edge over his opponent.

STATIC VISUAL ACUITY

It all starts with visual acuity. This very critical component of high performance vision is defined as the ability to resolve various sizes of letters or objects at various distances. It can be measured using a standard Snellen chart (see Figure 4.16), which yields the commonly heard vision readings of 20/20, 20/30, 20/50, etc. While this reading is not tremendously important in isolation, athletes should have at least 20/20 to 20/15 acuity in order to engage in most sporting activities. The level of static acuity with both eyes working together as a team should be better than that of each eye tested separately. The term "static" refers to measuring visual acuity while the athlete and the eye chart are stationary. For over two centuries, this examination has represented the baseline standard used to measure clarity of vision.

Deficits in static visual acuity can cause an inability to see and recognize small objects clearly and rapidly. No doubt, static visual acuity is important. Unfortunately, most sports involve movement. This is where dynamic visual acuity plays an even bigger role.

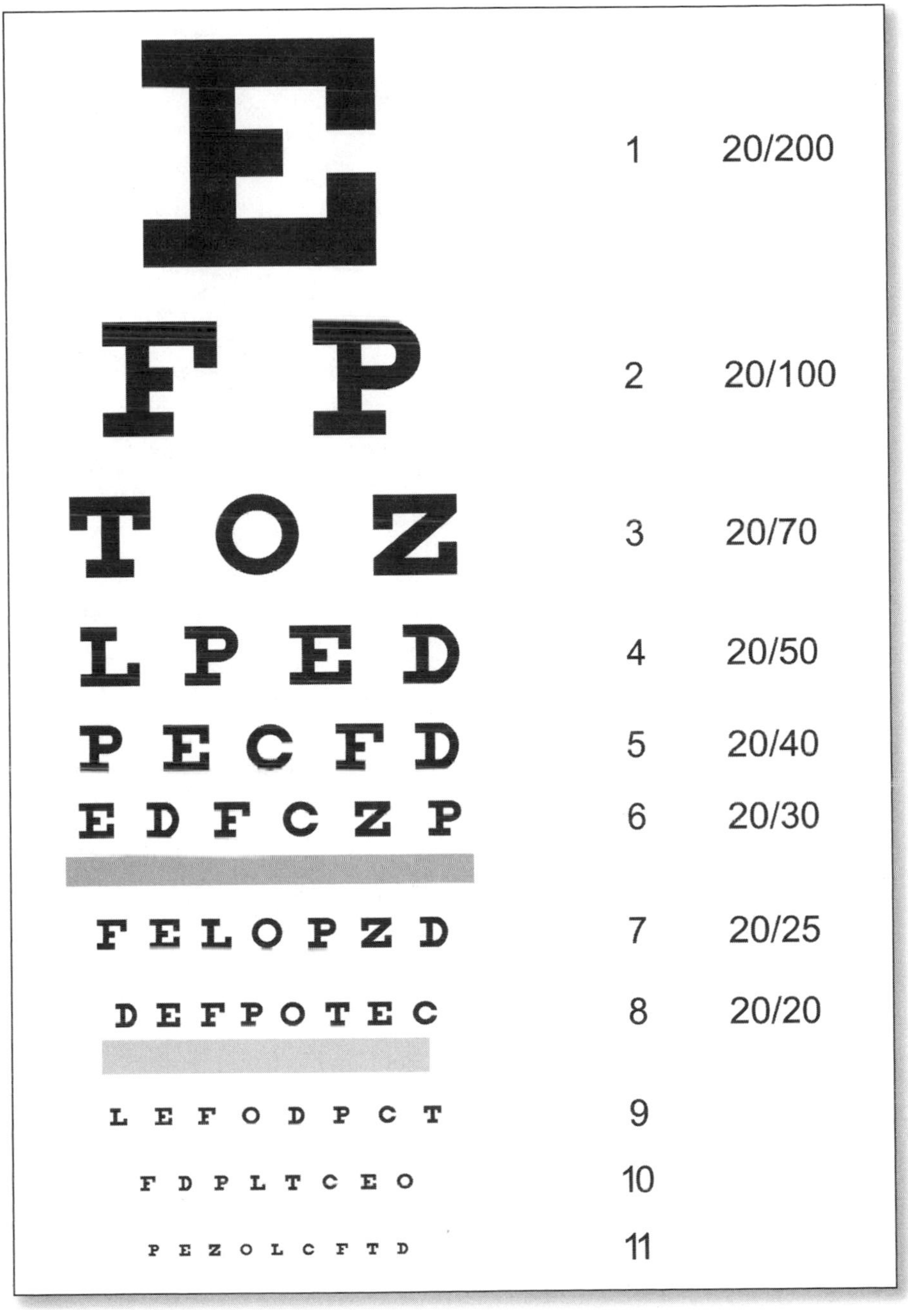

E	1	20/200
F P	2	20/100
T O Z	3	20/70
L P E D	4	20/50
P E C F D	5	20/40
E D F C Z P	6	20/30
F E L O P Z D	7	20/25
D E F P O T E C	8	20/20
L E F O D P C T	9	
F D P L T C E O	10	
P E Z O L C F T D	11	

Figure 4.16. Snellen Acuity Test

The standard eye chart developed by Herman Snellen in 1862 to quantify eyesight.

DYNAMIC VISUAL ACUITY

Most objects you see in the world are viewed in a dynamic manner. Generally, either the object or you are in motion. As a result, the act of seeing when motion is involved requires different and, perhaps, more demanding visual acumen than the act of viewing a stationary object. Problems with this skill can cause variable and inconsistent perception of an object being viewed. Fluctuation of clarity can affect timing, depth perception, object detail variation, and many other facets of good vision. Equipment designed to quantify a person's ability to maintain sharp vision when movement is introduced will likely play a valuable role in a complete high performance vision assessment.

VISUAL ADJUSTIBILITY

It is important to have a visual system that is flexible enough to adjust rapidly and guide the body's motor responses quickly and accurately in the face of changes in the surrounding environment. Adjustability is the art of being "tuned into" body responses, even though the demands of situations may vary. What is of critical importance is how long it takes your visual system to adjust to a changing environment, so that it may help guide the necessary responses to the outside world. A prime example is a racecar driver who must make instantaneous visual decisions as changes continue to occur along the track. Any deficit in this ability can slow the reactions of an athlete considerably, making any responses attempted unpredictable and inconsistent.

VISUAL CONCENTRATION

Visual concentration refers to the ability to focus attention on the athletic task at hand while filtering out peripheral distractions. Although humans may implement all five senses when trying to concentrate, by far the visual sense dominates in any quest to get in "the zone." In fact, 80 percent of concentration is visual. Athletes often employ stroboscopic lenses such as Sparq goggles or Impulse goggles, which create a visual distraction to train and push their abilities to concentrate to extreme levels. The lenses contain a special liquid crystal that becomes activated by a battery charge to create a stroboscopic flashing effect. In other words, they can be made to pulsate from totally opaque to completely clear according to set intervals. (Throw in a loud noise and the task becomes that much more affected by distraction, requiring even more concentration.) Athletes frequently report that their surroundings appear to be in slow motion upon completion of this very intense concentration technique. The ball or puck may also look dramatically larger.

VISUAL-MOTOR BALANCING SKILLS

The accuracy of shifting your body weight in reaction to a visual stimulus requires well-honed balance skills. Certainly, the inner ear (the vestibular system) plays a major role in achieving desirable

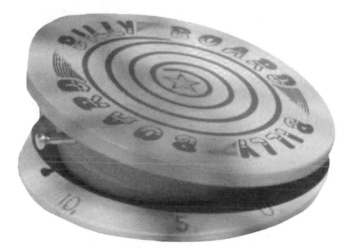

Figure 4.17. Billy Board

This balance board shifts according to the shifting weight of the test subject, who attempts to maintain balance while standing on the device.

results, but don't think that your eyes aren't equally important. Try standing on one foot for a few seconds. It is not that tough. Now shut your eyes and continue balancing on one foot. It is nearly impossible. During your visual-motor workup, certain instruments, including the Billy Board (see Figure 4.17), the Pro Fitter (see Figure 4.18), and the Wayne Balance Board (see Figure 4.19), may be used to assess your balance skills.

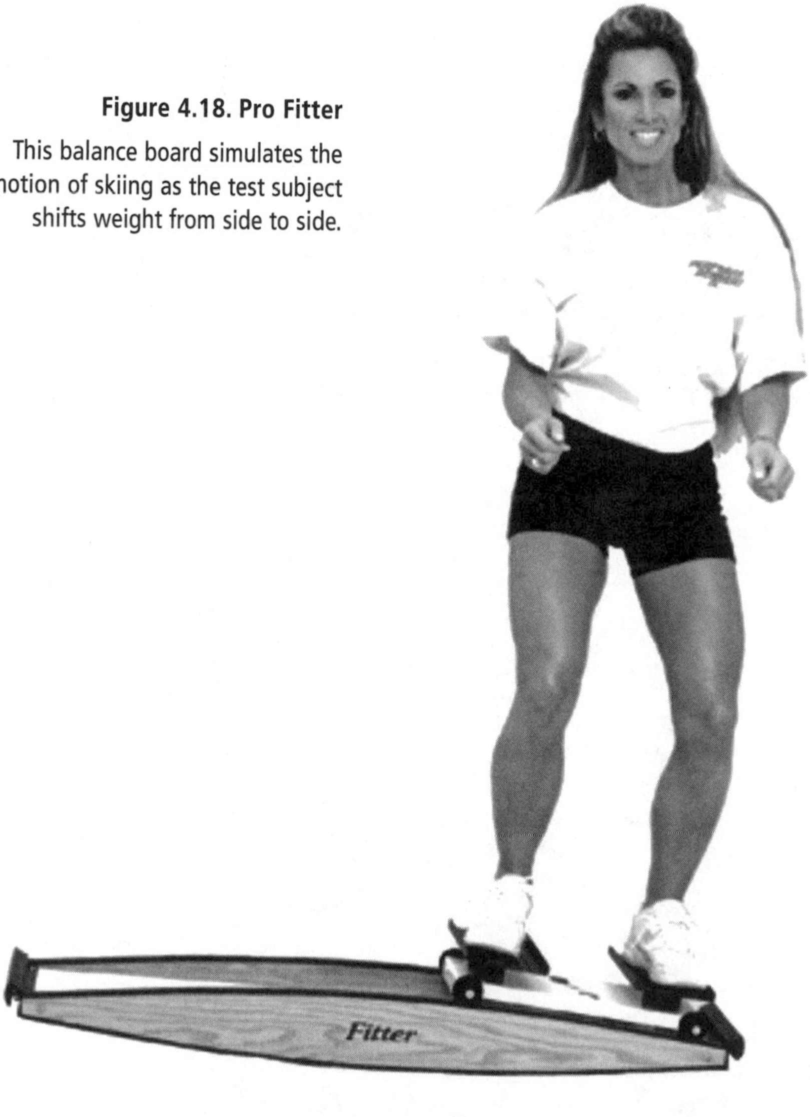

Figure 4.18. Pro Fitter

This balance board simulates the motion of skiing as the test subject shifts weight from side to side.

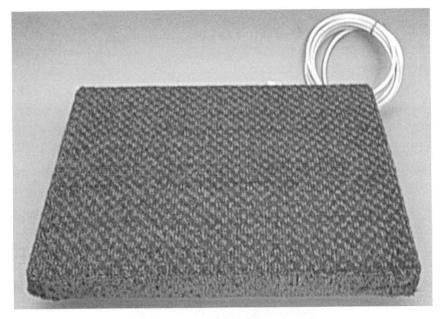

Figure 4.19. Wayne Balance Board

This balance board quantifies eye-to-foot balance when electronically connected to the Wayne Saccadic Fixator.

VISUALIZATION (POSITIVE IMAGERY)

Visualization may be defined as programming yourself for athletic success through the use of positive mental imaging. In essence, you are training your "mind's eye" to see yourself excelling in your chosen sport. By using the term "positive imagery," emphasis is placed on the importance of recalling and creating pictures that portray positive performance images in your brain. Your success may be greatly influenced by your mental attitude and muscle memory.

Visualization takes practice, as does any learned behavior. It is only through repetition that you may perfect your ability to train your "mind's eye" and program positive motor performance. Many superstars in the world of athletics attribute their competitive advantages to the ability to visualize effectively. This talent is an integral part of a good training program.

CONCLUSION

If you complete your high performance vision workup with a visual practitioner or trainer, you should be given a comprehensive report that includes a graph of strengths and weaknesses, as well as recommendations for initiating a systematic training program with your eye doctor or visual trainer. Your workup will include as many as thirty-five different visually driven categories rated on a sliding scale from excellent to poor. A report, however, is only as good as the game plan mapped out to maximize these many skills and put you on the road to excellence in your sport. Therefore, recommendations should be provided regarding how to get your eyes in gear for the athletic journey ahead of you. In Part Two of this book, you will learn numerous training techniques to help you succeed.

PART TWO

High Performance Vision Training

Part Two of this book shines a spotlight on the role of vision in sports. Once you understand the myriad ways in which the visual system impacts your ability to succeed athletically, you may then progress to training that system. High performance vision training includes a wide variety of exercises that may be performed at home, so you don't have to worry about making appointments or going out of your way to find a clinic. Should you decide to take the program a step further, high performance vision centers are available and offer training on technology that may be found only in an office setting.

Whether at home or in an office, you may also take advantage of visual-motor enhancement drills specific to your chosen sport, making your training even more beneficial. By putting all these elements together, you are sure to see positive results.

5.

The Role of Vision in Sports

It is perfectly reasonable to say that good vision is the most important skill to possess when it comes to playing sports. The basis of this idea rests in the knowledge that the visual system directs the motor system. The more quickly and accurately an athlete's visual system can process information, the better her chance of athletic success. For example, outstanding vision provides an athlete the ability to determine the nature of ball movement quickly. The eyes constantly monitor the flight of the ball, determining its spin, speed, and trajectory. The brain connects this visual information to motor-skill pathways to produce an appropriate physical response. Based on experience and an attention to detail, elite athletes can perceive the characteristics of a ball sooner than other players—a skill that allows these athletes to react faster and more accurately. Not all sports, of course, place the same visual demands on athletes, and the visual systems of players can differ greatly. A champion is one who understands her own visual abilities and knows how to use and improve them.

In an effort to assess overall vision, doctors and therapists rely on certain parameters, and visual enhancement may be achieved by developing abilities within these parameters. General principles of visual therapy include practice, feedback, measurement, difficulty level, and extrapolation of your data. You must continually perform the skill you are interested in improving, and this task must not be too easy or too difficult. You must also rely on a form of measurement to determine how well you are doing, of course, and you should be able to transfer your enhanced abilities to the athletic field or court.

ACCOMMODATION (FOCUSING FLEXIBILITY)

In many sports, the speed and accuracy with which you can shift your focus from near-field to far-field objects and back again play critical roles in success. For example, consider a table tennis player. The ball is constantly traveling back and forth across the net. The more proficient a player is in maintaining focus while following the ball, the more accurately the player will hit the ball. Athletes should begin training wearing their most accurate corrective lenses. In addition, they should begin training for distance—one eye at a time (monocular) initially, and eventually both eyes together (binocular).

ALIGNMENT

Think of your eyes as the two headlights of an automobile. If the beams align improperly on an object, you will misjudge the object's location and most assuredly fail in your efforts to accurately locate it in space. Conversely, if the beams align too far away from you, objects will appear to approach you more slowly. As a result, you'll react too late. When your eyes diverge excessively, the problem is called "exo posture."

ANTICIPATION TIMING

In many sports, the ability to predict the future location of a moving object (like a ball) is essential to athletic success. Whether the object is coming at you or traveling away from you, the goal is to time it right. Whatever your sport may be, there are training drills that can improve your anticipation timing.

CONTRAST SENSITIVITY (FINE DETAIL)

What is it that makes great athletes able to see the rotation of a baseball, the spin of a tennis ball, or the contours of a golf course? This extraordinary ability to interpret what we see with impeccable detail is known as outstanding contrast sensitivity.

Players commonly use the phrase "I'm seeing the ball really well" when they are in the proverbial "zone" of athletic achievement. These players are seeing the ball clearly and early, which slows down the game and makes athletic decisions easier to reach. On the flip side, a common complaint of many athletes is not being able to detect the ball in low-light situations. Many athletes perform well under daylight conditions but find great difficulty during nighttime games. The brain also controls the capacity to discern subtle differences at night. The brain may be trained to see more sharply and more clearly, but it may also be enhanced to work better in low-light environments.

DEPTH PERCEPTION

Seeing the world in stereo (stereopsis) is critical to athletic success in most sports. Try hitting a baseball or tennis ball with one eye closed! It's not easy to do! Depth perception flourishes when the eyes are capable of working together at an extremely high level. Fortunately, there are many ways to improve depth perception.

DYNAMIC VISUAL ACUITY

Most, if not all, sports involve motion. Whether the athlete or the ball is moving, there is a definite distinction between seeing clearly under conditions of motion and seeing clearly while sitting in a stationary position at an eye doctor's office and attempting to read a fixed eye chart. Obviously, motion makes tasks much more difficult. Any eye training drills that incorporate motion may be useful in enhancing dynamic visual acuity.

EYE TEAMING

The visual system of humans uses both eyes together as a team. The more the eyes are in sync with each other, the better the depth perception, and the greater the likelihood of making accurate spatial judgments. There are a number of simple exercises to train the eyes to work together at a higher level of proficiency.

EYE-TO-FOOT SPEED AND PATTERNING

An important skill in sports such as soccer and tennis, eye-to-foot speed and patterning refer to the coordination between an athlete's vision and movement of the feet. The most effective piece of equipment I have seen developed to enhance eye-to-foot quickness, agility, and patterning is the Quick Board, which will be discussed later on in this book. It allows you to increase raw foot speed, agility, and eye-to-foot reaction time, in addition to being a very portable aerobic running device. Whether at home or in a trainer's office, there are many drills you can do with the Quick Board.

EYE-TO-HAND-TO-FOOT-TO-BODY COORDINATION

Orchestrating the coordination between your eyes, your hands, your feet, and your body is no easy task. Yet great coordination is what separates the superstar from the rest of the pack. To a certain degree, this ability is a genetic gift that the greats are fortunate to have inherited. That being said, practice and repetition cannot be understated as key components to improving coordination. This neuromuscular programming can and does improve through practice.

EYE-TO-HAND SPEED

It is not only developing excellence in eye-hand coordination that counts, but also refining this skill with tremendous speed. So, how can you enhance your eye-to-hand speed? Like anything else, repetition and muscle memory play significant roles in improvement. A very popular way to work on eye-to-hand quickness these days would be to use any of the numerous sports simulators available on consoles such as the Nintendo Wii, the Microsoft X-Box, or the Sony PlayStation. These devices allow you to simulate the action in your sport while you are away from the playing field.

OCULAR MOTILITY

Ocular motility refer to smooth and efficient eye tracking movements. As you follow a moving object such as a ball or puck while under the pressures of a game, it can become a challenge to keep your eye on the ball smoothly. Pursuit movements refer to the smooth accurate movements of your eyes from point A to point B. As is the case with any skill, these eye tracking movements can improve with repetitive practice and ongoing effort.

PERIPHERAL AWARENESS

It is a God-given talent to recognize objects in the peripheral field of vision. Although the human peripheral field of vision is limited by anatomical boundaries, what separates the average athlete from the truly gifted one is an ability known as peripheral awareness. Although the human peripheral field is not adjustable, a person's peripheral awareness most definitely is.

SACCADES (JUMP FIXATIONS)

Many sports require rapid eye shifts from point A to point B to point C and so on. These shifts are known as "saccades," jump eye movements, or jump fixations. When performed quickly and accurately, these saccades can mean the difference between success and failure as an athlete.

SPEED OF RECOGNITION

As mentioned earlier, of all the senses, vision is by far the most dominant. In fact, the eyes process 80 percent of all sensory information that travels to the brain. Humans process this information very much like a computer. The eyes receive data much like a computer receives input. They then process it and transfer it to the brain, which is similar to a computer's memory system, where this information is stored until it is required to dictate a motor action or, in the case of a computer, output a result. So, it would behoove an athlete to complete this process as quickly and as accurately as possible. When training speed of recognition, a device called a tachistoscope is typically utilized.

SPEED OF RECOGNITION AND VISUAL MEMORY

Speed of recognition and visual memory may be described quite simply. The more information your eyes can absorb and transmit to your brain, the quicker your motor response will be, and the better you will play your game.

VISUAL CONCENTRATION

As 80 percent of sensory information comes from the eyes, making vision by far the dominant sense, it understandably follows that the eyes play an extremely dominant role in concentration.

VISUAL-MOTOR BALANCING SKILLS

Balance plays a vital role in many sports. When a golfer hits a drive, the momentum from the swing can easily throw her off balance. A diver on the edge of a diving board must have excellent balance before attempting a dive. The list of examples is endless. But what does balance have to do with the eyes? To answer this question, try the following task. Attempt to stand on one foot with your eyes open. It is not easy, but by no means is it impossible. Now try the same action with your eyes closed. I'd bet that most readers would remain standing only a matter of seconds. Later on in this book, you will read about drills to improve your balance. As with all these exercises, the idea is to create extreme conditions so that challenges in real situations become that much easier.

CONCLUSION

Before you embark on your high performance vision training program, I would like to clarify some basic rules. As you peruse the eye exercises described in the following chapters, you may note that some pieces of equipment are sophisticated and require the expertise of a certified doctor or trainer to operate. Do not be put off by this fact. You may do several of these drills and exercises quite easily on your own at home or on the playing field.

To truly benefit from this program, it is important to work not only on problem areas but also on all aspects of visual proficiency. Without a doubt, greater emphasis should be placed on weaker areas, but I must emphasize that whether you are a little leaguer, a weekend warrior, or an elite athlete, the intent of this program is to raise all facets of your vision and visual-motor skills to their maximum levels. To see results, I recommend practicing these skills three times a week for twenty minutes each time. Work on three or four diverse exercises each day and don't move on until you have perfected the skill you are attempting to develop.

6.

At-Home Eye Exercises

The beauty of high performance vision training is that there is more than one way to approach the program. To ensure you reap the maximum benefit available from your particular program, I would recommend you train with a doctor or trainer at a high performance vision facility. These centers have more sophisticated equipment, and much like a personal fitness trainer, they can monitor your progress and provide you with a more direct path towards taking your game to the next level. If this option is not practical for you, however, there are numerous drills and exercises that may be accomplished at home. If you opt for at-home training, I would urge you to follow the sequence of exercises in an order that will prevent you from attempting the difficult drills before you have perfected the easy ones.

HART CHART

This is certainly one of the exercises you can do at home on your own. It is designed to improve your accommodation ability, also known as focus flexibility. A Hart Chart is nothing more than a random sequence of letters arranged in rows and columns on a standard sheet of paper (US letter size) to be displayed on a wall at a distance of ten feet. It may be made at home, printed from online sources, or purchased from Bernell Corporation (www.bernell.com). When training near focus, a miniature Hart Chart is also necessary.

Post the chart of letters on a wall about ten feet away. With your handheld card of letters at typical reading length (about sixteen inches), read the first line of small letters aloud. Now focus on the wall and read the first row of letters again. Focus back on the small letters in your hand and read the second row. Keep switching back and forth, one row at a time. Do the exercise with one eye open and the other eye covered by your hand or a patch, and then switch eyes. Switch back to the first eye, but this time move the card one inch closer to your eye for every row of letters you read on the small card. Repeat with the other eye. Finally, perform the exercise with both eyes open at a reading distance of sixteen inches. Make certain all letters read are crystal clear. If they are not, you are too far from the wall or the handheld chart is too close. Undertake these sessions five times a week for ten to fifteen minutes each time. Doing this exercise every once in a while will not be of any help.

RED-GREEN ACCOMMODATIVE ROCK

This exercise is also meant to improve accommodation and is an extension of the focus flexibility training procedure described in the previous section. This test is administered in the same manner, except the charts are covered with a transparent filter that alternates between red and green. When special red-green lenses are worn during this exercise, the goal is not only to boost focus speed but also to avoid the potential obstacle of having one eye shut down during the training process. The red-green lenses and red-green filter force both eyes to participate together, ensuring binocularity. Red-green filter cards and glasses may also be obtained from Bernell Corporation. (See Figure 6.1.)

VISUAL TRACINGS

Designed to develop ocular motility, this task has a simple goal. Using a timer, the participant is required to keep his head as still as possible while tracking the twisted lines from start to finish as

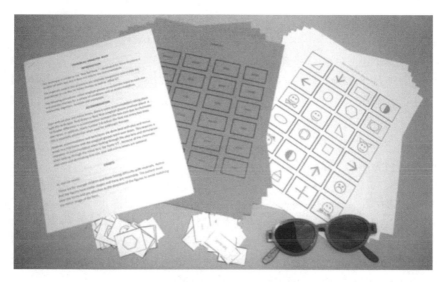

Figure 6.1. Franzblau Red-Green Anaglyph Rock

Wearing red-green lenses, the test subject views a series of special cards
to train focus flexibility and force both eyes to work together.

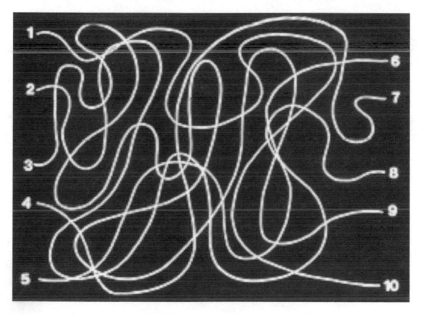

Figure 6.2. Visual Tracings

The goal of this display of wavy lines intersecting on a board is to determine
where each line starts and finishes using only your eyes.

quickly as he can. (See Figure 6.2.) You may start out wearing an eye patch on one eye. Work on improving your pursuit eye movements while keeping your head as steady as possible (try balancing a book on your head) and tracking the wavy lines from start to finish. Advance from one eye at a time to both eyes together once you have mastered the first method.

FLASHLIGHT TAG

Another method of enhancing ocular motility, this exercise may be practiced at home with a trainer or friend. Have your partner stand behind you in a relatively dark room and shine a flashlight beam onto the wall in front of you. Superimpose your own flashlight beam on top of your partner's without moving your head. The goal is to keep your light on top of the other light as your partner's beam moves left, right, up, down, diagonally, and in a circular path. This training exercise becomes more difficult if you use a smaller light, such as a penlight.

MARSDEN BALL

The Marsden Ball is another great tool to improve ocular motility. To make a Marsden Ball, drill a hole through a tennis ball-sized sponge ball. Take a cord of about four feet in length and thread it through the ball. Secure the string with a knot and hang the ball from the ceiling. (If you create a pulley system, you can change the height of the ball to adjust it to your eye level.) With different colored markers, write letters and numbers all over the ball. You now have a Marsden Ball. (See Figure 6.3.)

Swing the ball in any of five possible directions (left to right, right to left, forward and back, diagonally, or circularly) and call out the letters or numbers on the ball while it is in motion. The goal is to keep your head as still as possible, forcing your eyes to do the work exclusively. You may want to balance a book on your head at first to prevent excessive head movement. If you'd like to add an

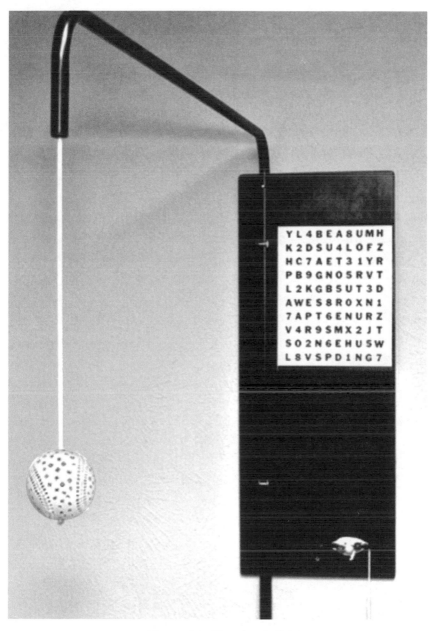

Figure 6.3. Marsden Ball

This ball has letters and numbers randomly placed on its surface. As it swings, the test subject must call out the letters and numbers seen. The test subject's head must remain stationary during this exercise.

extra layer of difficulty, put three stripes, each of a different color, on a rolling pin. While balancing on a balance board, attempt to call out the letters or numbers while bunting the ball with a specific stripe on the rolling pin.

PEGBOARD ROTATOR

You can either purchase a pegboard rotator or make a simplified version of this device by fashioning a pegboard into a ten-inch diameter circle and mounting it on a turntable. (See Figure 6.4.) The object is to insert golf tees one at a time into the holes of the spinning disc without moving your head. The trick is to lock your vision onto one hole, pursue it with your eyes only, and anticipate its location to insert the tee accurately. You can expect to track the center-most holes most easily. Moving your focus towards the rim of the disc makes the holes much tougher to follow.

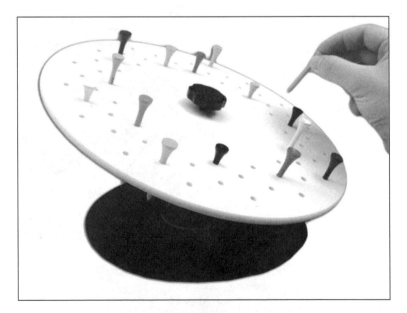

Figure 6.4. Pegboard Rotator

This disc has small holes and rotates at variable speed. The test subject must place a golf tee into a particular hole while keeping a steady head.

THE DOMINANT EYE

As discussed earlier, we are all born with a dominant, or preferred, eye. In the act of seeing, one eye always leads and the other eye always follows. In one study of Canadian hockey players, it was found that the dominant eye processes information to the brain fourteen milliseconds faster than the non-dominant eye. That might not sound like much, but in fast-moving situations such as stopping a puck or hitting a baseball, fourteen milliseconds can mean the difference between making a successful save or not, or getting a base hit or not.

Your eyes never look at the exact same point in space. The dominant eye aims precisely on the object of regard while the other eye aims slightly off line. This very unique phenomenon creates an overlap of eye positioning that produces three-dimensional vision. Simply put, if both eyes aimed at exactly the same place, you would be able to see objects only in two dimensions, or flat. Similarly, you have a dominant hand and foot, unless you are ambidextrous.

As previously described, to determine your dominant eye, fixate on a small object at a distance (greater than eight feet away). For example, this can be a doorknob or any small object at eye level. Extend both arms fully in front of you while forming a small triangular opening between your two hands. Set the sight of your object of regard through the triangle and then shut one eye at a time.

Observe which eye's line of vision remains on the doorknob. This is your dominant eye. Your dominant hand is the one with which you write, although this may vary in some cases. (For example, some left-handed people write with their right hands, having been encouraged to do so as children. Studies have shown, however, that when hand dominance is forcibly altered in childhood, there is an increased risk of inducing a stuttering problem.) In addition, an ambidextrous person may be right-handed when writing but left-handed when throwing a ball, swinging a bat, shooting a puck, or performing some other sporting task. When it comes to feet, a simple way to assess the dominant foot is to place a ball (a soccer ball will do, but any size ball will work) in front of you on the ground, instinctively walk up to it, and kick it. When this action is done without thinking, the foot you chose to do the kicking is your dominant or preferred foot.

Can eye dominance be switched through training? The answer is unconditionally no. As mentioned, any attempt to change a person's eye dominance may result in stuttering issues, reading confusion, or coordination problems. The better approach is to teach the athlete to be aware of her dominant eye and the role it plays in visual decision making. For example, a left-eyed batter who also bats with his left hand would be advised to turn his head so that his dominant eye faces the pitcher more directly.

BUILDING CONVERGENCE

In order to strengthen eye alignment, you must work on building convergence. There is an easily performed at-home exercise to do just that. Hold out your two index fingers at about arm's length, one directly in front of the other. Fixate your eyes on the fingernail of the nearest finger and slowly bring it closer in your line of sight. As your hand moves closer, the finger at the greater distance (the one you are not focusing on) will appear to split into a double image. Continue to bring the closer finger towards your nose until the fingernail you are focusing on divides into two images. Slowly move the closer finger back to its original position and repeat this exercise several times. (See Figure 6.5.)

BUILDING DIVERGENCE

Another way to improve eye alignment is to build divergence. Cover one eye and use the other to focus on a pencil held at arm's length directly ahead of you. Keeping your head facing straight ahead, slowly move your arm towards the side. Follow the pencil with your open eye until it disappears from view. Repeat this exercise several times with each eye.

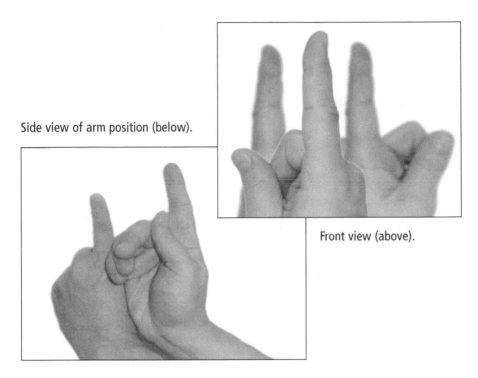

Side view of arm position (below).

Front view (above).

Figure 6.5. Building Convergence

The test subject moves his index finger slowly towards his nose, attempting
to continue seeing it as one finger while the demand on both eyes to maintain fixation
becomes more and more intense.

LIFESAVER CARD

Lifesaver Cards may be easily purchased online and can help improve eye teaming. (See Figure 6.6.) Once you've acquired a Lifesaver Card, position a pencil about twelve inches away from your eyes, making sure it is set between your eyes. Hold the Lifesaver Card behind the pencil at arm's length. While viewing the tip of the pencil, attempt to merge the bottom two Lifesavers together into one Lifesaver (a combined red-green color). Be aware of the words "CLEAR THESE WORDS" on the bottom Lifesaver while continuing to focus on the pencil tip. Attempt to remove the pencil while keeping the bottom two Lifesavers merged as one.

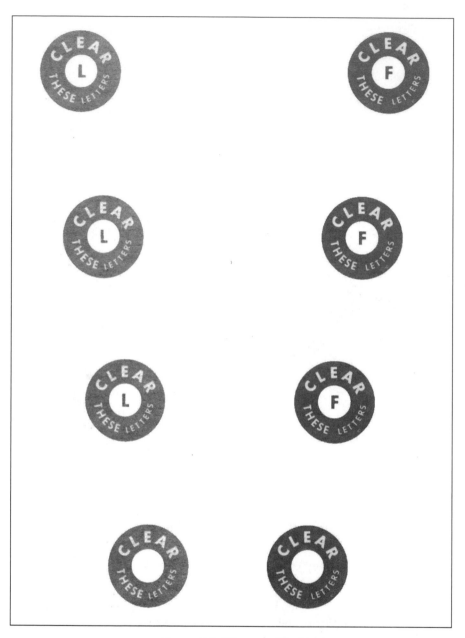

Figure 6.6. Lifesaver Card

This simple handheld card is used to build eye-muscle strength and eye-teaming ability. The test subject allows the eyes to create an imaginary third circle situated in between the two circles being viewed.

BULL'S-EYE CARD

Another eye-teaming exercise involves the use of a Bull's-Eye Card (see Figure 6.7), which involves a task similar to that associated with the Lifesaver Card. Hold the Bull's-Eye Card at arm's length. Use a pencil held in front of the Bull's-Eye Card to assist you in merging the two bull's-eyes into one image. Remove the pencil and observe the floating circles, the letters "A" and "B" on the bottom of the card, and the word "CLEAR."

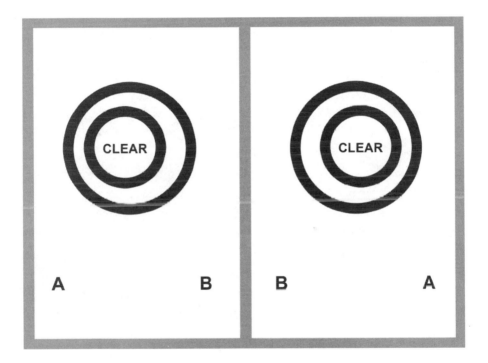

Figure 6.7. Bull's-Eye Card

This training device improves the ability of the eyes to work as a team. The test subject holds two cards at arm's length and attempts to merge the two bull's-eyes into a virtual bull's-eye that appears to float in space in three dimensions.

ULTIMEYES GABOR CONTRAST TARGETS

Recently, an innovative computer software program called Ultimeyes was introduced to train the brain to see clearer and sharper. Dedicated to the improvement of contrast sensitivity and fine detail, ULTIMEYES is especially helpful to those who play in low-light environments, as it trains the brain to maximize edge detection. The app itself is interactive and combines vision, hearing, and touch to create a multisensory environment that produces marked visual improvement. (See Figure 6.8.)

The ULTIMEYES workout consists of players interacting with the app four times weekly for thirty sessions, each session lasting about twenty to twenty-five minutes. Each session tests vision prior to training and customizes training for the user during that session. The athlete being trained is asked to view a computer screen at a distance of no less than eight feet. He is then shown randomly changing line gradient patterns known as Gabor Targets, which appear fainter as the screens change sequentially. He is asked to use a computer mouse to click on the randomly positioned targets as they appear. This task increases in difficulty with each successive screen change.

In essence, this workout teaches the visual cortex (the most sensitive component of sight recognition in the brain) to increase its ability to make use of the macula (the central dot that sits on the retina and is needed for highly critical central vision). Neuroscientists have proven that the brain has a tremendously high level of neuroplasticity, or flexibility, allowing it to accomplish such skills as finely tuned eyesight. This type of training pushes the brain to make it see better as opposed to treating the aspects of vision provided only by the eyes.

Although ULTIMEYES has not been studied for very long, related studies of the brain suggest its results can last for years. Occasional training (once a week or once monthly) may be necessary to maintain these positive outcomes. Repetition, attention, and a scientifically proven program are keys to vision enhancement. This software is available through the company's website (www.ultimeyesvision .com) and is also offered as an app on iTunes.

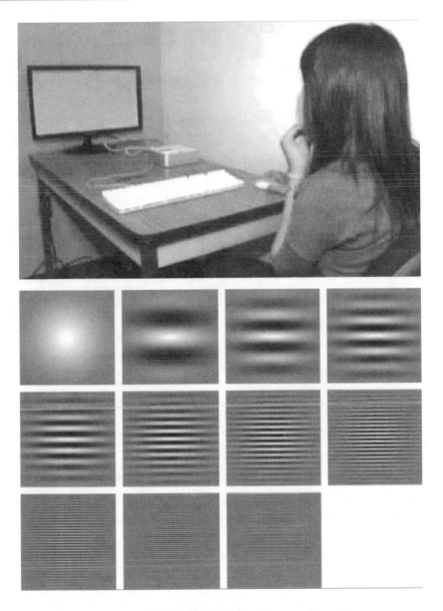

Figure 6.8. ULTIMEYES Gabor Contrast Targets

This test involves randomly presented images of horizontal gradient lines called Gabor Targets viewed on a computer screen from a minimum of eight feet away. The test subject attempts to find these targets, using a computer mouse to click on them to confirm the ability to see them.

POINTER AND STRAW

Meant to boost depth perception, the pointer and straw exercise may be easily attempted from the comfort of your own home. With a pointer, or common pick-up stick, and an ordinary drinking straw, attempt to feed the stick through the straw at varied distances from your eyes. (See Figure 6.9.) Try to accomplish this task while altering the position of the straw (i.e., holding the straw vertically, horizontally, or diagonally).

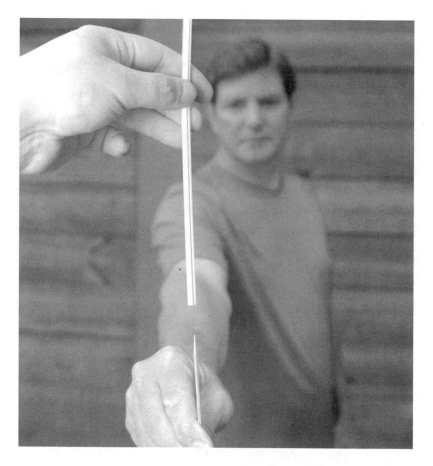

Figure 6.9. Pointer and Straw

The test subject attempts to place a pointer into a straw without hitting the walls of the straw.

HEEL-TOE AND DISTANCE ESTIMATION

Depth perception may also be improved by practicing this heel-toe exercise at home. Select an object across the room and predict how many heel-to-toe paces you will need to make to reach that object. Pace off the distance accurately by walking heel-to-toe until you get there.

Spatial awareness and depth perception may also be developed by having someone (your trainer or a friend) place two objects at different distances and ask you to state which object is closer than the other. Have your trainer or friend alter the distance at which the two objects are standing every few guesses.

ANTICIPATION TIMING DRILL

The anticipation timing drill is a training exercise that can improve your anticipation timing. Close your eyes and do not open them until you are given a signal to do so. For example, at the crack of the bat, open your eyes to anticipate the flight of the baseball in time to field it efficiently. Or, at the sound of the tennis racquet striking the ball, open your eyes and move to return the serve. Or, at the sound of a specific hiking cadence number, open your eyes to track the flight of the pass to you while being covered by a defender. There are numerous variations of this task.

Next, try turning your back away from the sporting task. On a specific signal, turn around and complete the athletic requirement at hand. Finally, complete the skills listed above while initially lying on your back and getting up quickly to react at the sound of a specific signal. The Bassin Anticipation Timer is an outstanding training device that can enhance your ability to anticipate the position of a moving object dramatically. Repetition on this instrument can really improve your muscle memory to accomplish these varied anticipation exercises successfully.

QUICK BOARD

Available for purchase online (www.thequickboard.com), this device may be used at home just as easily as it is used in a professional's office to train eye-to-foot speed and patterning. The Quick Board consists of a rectangular floor board with five yellow circles distributed in a pattern. Each circle is electronically foot-touch sensitive and sends a signal to an electronic tablet positioned in front of the board on a tripod. (See Figure 6.10.)

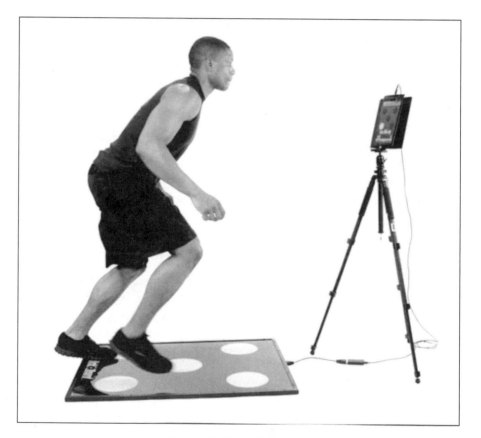

Figure 6.10. Quick Board

The test subject runs specific patterns on this electronic board as quickly and accurately as possible to measure and train eye-foot coordination, visual-motor sequencing skills, and raw foot speed.

Three Quick Board drills are useful as part of your high per-formance vision program. The first one trains raw foot speed. The tablet records the number of repetitions achievable in a ten-second span as the athlete being trained rapidly switches feet back and forth on the two circles at the front. Several accomplished soccer players have been known to register close to 150 repetitions during this drill. Breaking 100 is an optimistic goal for the weekend warrior. The second drill trains visual-motor sequencing. The athlete is asked to run a pattern on the board, starting with the left foot touch-ing the upper left circle followed by the right foot landing on the upper right circle. Next, the left foot travels to the lower left circle. Finally, the right foot lands on the lower right circle. This sequence is repeated as many times as possible over a ten-second time frame. A goal of thirty complete cycles is considered excellent. Lastly, the third drill works on eye-to-foot coordination. When the timer begins, five yellow squares begin to light up individually on the tablet. The athlete is required to place a foot on the circle that corre-sponds to the illuminated square on screen. Over a ten-second period, a score of ten or greater would be considered good.

BALANCE BOARD

You can enhance your eye-to-hand-to-foot-to-body coordination at home by using an easy-to-build balance board. Purchase a 3/4-inch thick 2 x 2 plywood board from a local lumberyard. In addition, get five 1 1/4-inch flathead wood screws and a piece of medium coarse sandpaper. You will also need a saw, a drill, and a screwdriver. Cut a 16-inch square, a 4-inch square, and a 3-inch square from the plywood. Attach the 4-inch square to the center of the largest square using the four wood screws. Attach the remaining 3-inch square to the 4-inch square using the remaining wood screw. Sand the edges and you have a balance board!

Next, take a large white poster board and draw sixteen bold arrows on it. (See Figure 6.11.) Attach the board to a wall about eight feet away or farther. While on the balance board, with the help of the

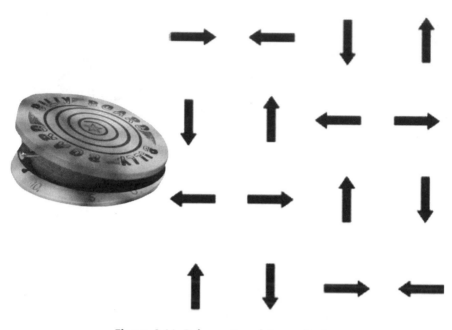

Figure 6.11. Balance Board Arrow Poster

The arrows on this poster board guide the test subject to shift her weight
on a balance board correspondingly.

beat of a metronome, shift your body weight to match the direction
of the arrows on each line. As you improve in this task, increase the
speed of the metronome and change the direction in which you read
the arrows (vertically, diagonally, or around the perimeter).

GOLF DRILL

Here's an exercise that will boost your eye-to-hand-to-foot-to-body
coordination and allow your eyes to guide your hands to strike a
golf ball precisely. When lining up the ball on the tee or putting
green, focus on a piece of the ball rather than on the entire ball. With
your dominant eye on the ball, position the logo of the ball so that
it is in the direction of the shot at the desired point of contact on the
ball's surface. Tell your "mind's eye" that the logo will remain in
place exactly as it has been set even after you have struck the ball.

TENNIS DRILL

Eye-to-hand-to-foot-to-body coordination may also be improved by practicing this tennis drill. Take a standard tennis ball and with a color felt marker put four large circles (approximately one inch in diameter) on different surfaces of the ball. Repeat this action with other tennis balls using a different color for the circles placed on each ball. Your challenge is to call out the particular color of these circles on the ball being hit to you before the ball contacts your racquet. The goal here is to teach you to follow the ball all the way to the racquet. This drill also trains tennis players to stay closed in their backhand strokes.

OFF THE WALL

Here's a great way to fine-tune your eye-to-hand-to-foot-to-body coordination and enhance your quickness. Have your trainer stand behind you as you face a wall. Stand approximately five feet from the wall looking straight ahead. At the verbal signal "NOW," your trainer should toss a ball against the wall. Your task is to catch the ball. To increase the level of difficulty, you could catch the ball after one bounce while standing farther than five feet away. You could start even closer than five feet from the wall and use a large ball, such as a volleyball, and then work your way up to catching a small ball, such as a Super Ball.

PERIPHERAL WALL CHART

Set up an 8 x 11 piece of paper horizontally and create a sequence of letters (or numbers or a mix of both). (See Figure 6.12.) With the chart on a wall at eye level, focus your eyes on the small "x" in the center of the piece of paper. Using your peripheral vision, identify the grouping of letters surrounding the small "x." Work your way out to the most peripheral letters while always keeping your eyes focused on the central "x."

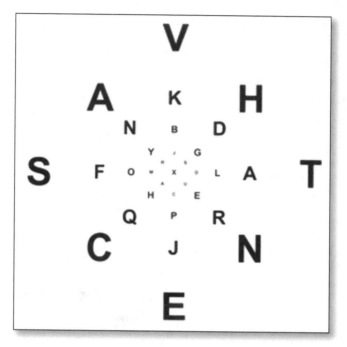

Figure 6.12. Peripheral Wall Chart

This pattern of letters progresses from the center of vision to the periphery
to improve peripheral awareness.

PERIPHERAL OBSERVATION

A simple drill that you can work on with absolutely no equipment involves fixating on an object in front of you while attempting to identify objects in the periphery, thus training your peripheral awareness. Over the years, I have instructed professional athletes to practice this skill while waiting at airports for their flights to arrive. Strive to increase this expansion of peripheral awareness to more extreme angles over time.

RULER PERIPHERAL TRAINING

Another method of increasing your peripheral awareness is to take a standard twelve-inch ruler and write a small letter or number on one end of it (about one inch from the edge). In a sitting position while fixating on an object at eye level across the room (e.g., a doorknob), attempt to see the letter or number on the end of the ruler clearly as you slowly move it in an arc into your periphery. When you reach your limit, move the ruler slightly back into sight and attempt to expand your range once again. Try this exercise with the ruler moving in an arc to the right, to the left, at different angles, with both eyes open, and with one eye open.

PRE-MADE FLASH CARDS

To work on your speed of recognition and visual memory, you can photograph scenes depicting a sporting action such as a pitcher's arm releasing a specific pitch. Have your trainer show you these action scenes for a fraction of a second and then ask you to name as quickly as you can the type of pitch and the hand with which the pitcher is throwing the ball.

SIMPLE CONCENTRATION TECHNIQUE

As with most endeavors in life, the ability to concentrate well is crucial in regard to athletic achievement. To boost your visual concentration, focus on an object—for example, the letter "S" on the logo on a Spalding basketball. Maintain your view of the ball and relax. If your attention wanders, return it to the letter "S." Address the quality of concentration rather than on the length of time you're able to stay focused. Begin with only a minute or two, take a brief break, and then return your attention to your chosen object. Continue alternately focusing and relaxing for ten to twenty minutes. Increase the length of time you focus only as the strength of your concentration grows. Be sure not to compromise the quality of attention for the quantity of time.

As your training continues, you'll feel your concentration acquiring a laser-like intensity. You may then gradually increase the length of time of focused attention.

CONCLUSION

As we all know, every athlete is forever seeking a competitive edge. Most of us would agree that our eyes play an enormous role in achieving that edge. What makes high performance vision training great is that it allows you to improve your visual-cognitive motor skills through the use of sophisticated equipment found only in specialty clinics and training centers, but also makes it possible to train at home and on the playing field. There is a wide variety of exercises and drills that can start you on your way to great vision without forcing you to leave your own neighborhood. Of course, if you wish to experience the entire spectrum of exercises associated with high performance vision training, a visit to a professional remains an option.

7.

In-Office Eye Exercises

Studies have shown that baseball players tend to possess better vision than those who do not play this sport. Is this because athletes with good vision naturally gravitate towards baseball? Do baseball players have fewer problems with vision? The answer to both questions is no. Since athletes and non-athletes have similar vision problems requiring optical correction (glasses, contact lenses, LASIK), the basis of this statistic is not to be found only in the optics of the eye but also in brain function. Players in sports such as baseball simply develop their good vision. The repetitive viewing of a baseball at long distances enhances the brain's ability to see.

Vision is a combination of optics and brain capability. In fact, in a major research study, brain training improved a college baseball team's vision by over 30 percent, leading to a higher team batting average and more team wins. Additionally, in 2011, brain-trained vision improvements helped Casey Kotchman to his finest season in professional baseball. There is no doubt that the right training regimen can improve brain capability and enable the individual undergoing training to see more clearly.

While many high performance vision exercises may be performed at home, there are a number of vision-enhancing devices and tools that are generally found only in a specialist's office. If you are able to take advantage of the services offered by a vision specialist, in-office training can lead to positive and significant results.

LOOSE LENS ROCK

The idea behind this exercise is to create flexibility in the focusing lenses of the eyes, which should result in enhanced accommodation. These loose lenses are designed at different strengths and can produce magnification (plus) or minification (minus) power. By alternating between each power level while viewing an object at a distance, the individual forces the lenses of the eyes to flex back and forth, increasing their elasticity. This improvement in elasticity allows athletes to make rapid decisions in sports that require instant shifts in focus from far-field to near-field and vice versa.

ACCOMMODATIVE FLIPPERS

Instead of loose lenses, your high performance vision specialist may provide you with a series of binocular lens flippers known as accommodative flippers (see Figure 4.12), which can facilitate the shifts in focus described in the last section. These flippers can help you achieve the same goal of lens elasticity.

SMI EYE TRACKING GLASSES

The SMI Eye Tracking Glasses and their corresponding recording unit (see Figure 7.1) make up the latest version of a high-tech eye-tracking device used to improve ocular motility. This apparatus allows an athlete to evaluate and perfect the alignment of his dominant eye as he sets his sight on an object. The computer recording of the position of gaze is demonstrated with the help of a blue Lifesaver target, which coincides with the position of the dominant eye. Access to this training device is a good reason to visit a high performance vision specialist, although it is available for purchase should you so choose.

NEUROTRACKER

Thanks to 3D technology, NeuroTracker (see Figure 7.2 and Figure 7.3) trains ocular motility, enhancing visual-cognitive performance

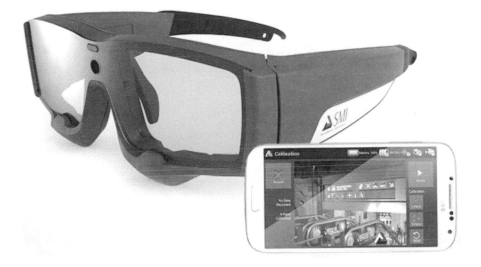

Figure 7.1. SMI Eye Tracker

These specialized glasses track and record the position of the eyes
as they fixate on an object.

in sports. NeuroTracker is a system that measures and trains awareness and attention in athletes of all ages. Awareness and attention
are the key mental skills that allow athletes to make better decisions on the field. NeuroTracker training takes place in an immer-
sive 3D environment, which stimulates the brain in a way that taps
into an athlete's mental ability. The benefits of NeuroTracker are
founded on science both in the laboratory and on the playing field.
In fact, NeuroTracker is so fundamental to sport training that users
who improve their NeuroTracker scores also demonstrate better
overall performance on the field. This is certainly why more and
more elite teams are using NeuroTracker as one of their premier
tools for scouting athletic talent.

Research studies across a wide number of sports show time and
again that the main difference between elite athletes and average
athletes is mental performance, not physical prowess. Instead of
training an individual for a particular play, NeuroTracker hones
cognitive tools in a way that may be of benefit in any sporting

situation. This is similar to the effect of doing squats, an exercise that improves sprint acceleration and vertical leap, skills that are advantageous in a wide variety of sports.

Using your visual system, NeuroTracker isolates the core mental elements of awareness and attention and trains them intensively. According to Kathleen Duffy, Director of Neuromedical Business Development for NeuroTracker, a typical training session is short and simple to do, but still a challenging task. Athletes focus on four of eight targets moving through a 3D environment. They must maintain mental focus at high speeds. Using classic training principles—isolation, overload, repetition—NeuroTracker allows athletes to train the mental skills that lead to success in sports. Players who train with a vision specialist with NeuroTracker may process visual

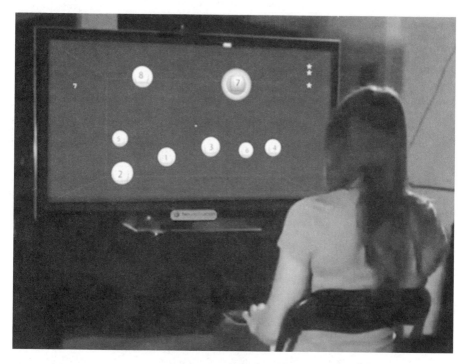

Figure 7.2. NeuroTracker

This 3D projection system trains the test subject to process the position
of multiple targets quickly and accurately.

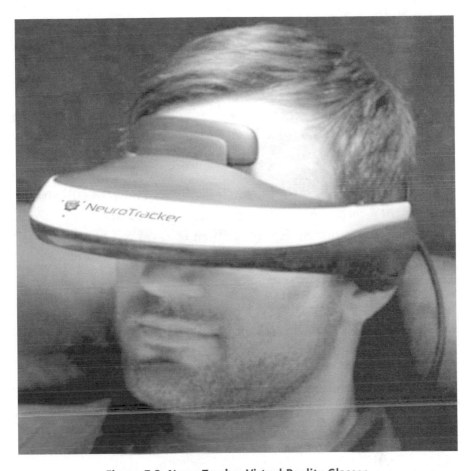

Figure 7.3. NeuroTracker Virtual Reality Glasses

This apparatus projects images of NeuroTracker multisensory targets onto the eyes of the test subject.

information more quickly and read movement more effectively. They may also be better at resisting mental fatigue.

When your high performance vision specialist talks about improving your vision, she is not actually talking about your eyes, per se, but rather about your visual system, which refers to how your brain sees, interprets, and processes the millions of visual cues on the playing field. NeuroTracker trains your visual system to give you the competitive edge required for athletic success.

THE KING-DEVICK TEST

Developed by Dr. Alan King and Dr. Steven Devick in 1976, this simple test is easy to administer and has been a proven indicator of oculomotor deficiency regarding saccadic eye movement. In fact, published medical studies have determined that inabilities revealed by the King-Devick test (see Figure 7.4) are an indicator of mild traumatic brain injury (TBI) or concussion after head trauma.

The King-Devick test is an objective method of evaluating visual tracking and saccadic eye movement. It is based on the time taken to perform rapid number naming. It involves reading aloud a series of single digit numbers from left to right on three test cards. The

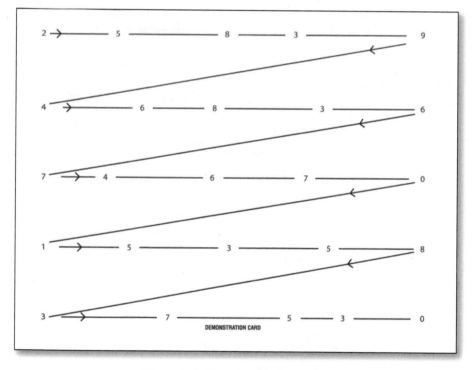

Figure 7.4. King-Devick Test Card

This tracking test is used to detect poor oculomotor skills, which may relate to deficits in reading ability in school children or signal a possible concussion in an athlete.

participant is asked to read the numbers on each card from left to right as quickly and as accurately as possible. The test taker is scored on each test, with the sum of the three tests constituting the final result.

A newer version of this eye-tracking test called the Developmental Eye Movement (DEM) test was developed by Dr. Jack Richman and is now available. Both tracking tools are very useful in screening for concussion and traumatic brain injury.

WAYNE SACCADIC FIXATOR AND VMET

Athletes may train jump fixation eye movement using the Wayne Saccadic Fixator (see Figure 7.5), which is a device that features three concentric circles of lights around a center light. With the square panel mounted on a wall, the patient attempts to touch the lights as they are illuminated randomly. The goal is to hit as many light targets as possible during a predetermined time period.

The Visual Motor Enhancement Trainer, or VMET (see Figure 7.6), uses actual background scenes of relevant sporting events to test and train eye-hand coordination and tracking skill. Patients are asked to identify small targets that change position on the screen and accurately touch them as quickly and efficiently as possible. The targets will continue to change position and may be sped up.

SENAPTEC SENSORY STATION

Athletes who are more capable at processing sensory information are often better than their peers. Measuring sensory-motor strengths and weaknesses is a critical part of athlete screening and training. While some people naturally have better visual skills, it is possible to improve visual and sensory-motor abilities. The Senaptec Sensory Station accomplishes this task by evaluating athletes and developing vision enhancement programs for them. This device even provides ways to track improvement and further refine sensory-motor skills.

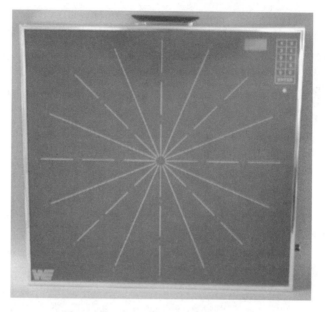

Figure 7.5. Wayne Saccadic Fixator

This electronic device is used in numerous testing and training regimens
to improve an array of visual-cognitive motor skills.

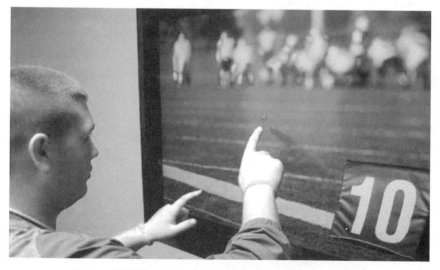

Figure 7.6. Visual Motor Enhancement Trainer (VMET)

This tool uses a screen whose display can be programmed to correspond to
a variety of realistic sporting activities to test and train eye-hand coordination.

The Senaptec Sensory Station measures ten visual and sensory-motor skills: visual clarity, contrast sensitivity, depth perception, near-far quickness, target capture, perception span, multiple object tracking, peripheral target response, go and no-go, and reaction time. These assessments are based on reliable, valid, and well-established methods described in peer-reviewed literature.

Once an athlete's evaluation has been completed, the Senaptec Sensory Station provides an immediate comparison to her peer population. This report allows for the most meaningful identification of an athlete's sensory performance strengths and, more importantly, the opportunities for continued enhancement. The Senaptec Sensory Station produces an athlete-specific training enhancement plan as part of the detailed analysis generated.

STROBE TRAINING

Strobe training may be used to hone eye-to-hand-to-foot-to-body coordination. The intermittent states of brightness and darkness created by the strobe light (or specially designed strobe-effect eyeglasses) challenge the individual to maintain concentration in the face of demanding athletic challenges. The goal is to start with a reasonably rapid flash. As training progresses, the individual should attempt to reach higher performance benchmarks at slower intervals between darkness and brightness. The slower the intervals, the tougher the task becomes. It is important to note, however, that strobe lights may cause epileptic seizures in people who are predisposed to this condition.

WAYNE PERIPHERAL AWARENESS TRAINER (PAT)

Designed by Wayne Engineering, the company behind the Wayne Saccadic Fixator, the Wayne Peripheral Awareness Trainer, or Wayne PAT, has a variety of drills to improve peripheral awareness. Consult with a high performance vision expert near you to customize a program for your particular sport.

One PAT drill requires you to fixate on a central red light as peripheral lights appear randomly one at a time. Your task is to direct a joystick in the same direction as the peripheral light until it disappears and moves to a different zone in your periphery. The wrinkle is to program the central red light to turn on and off randomly. You are permitted to shift the joystick only when the central red light is illuminated. If you shift it when the central red light is off, your final score will be penalized.

TACHISTOSCOPIC IMAGES

Training speed of recognition may be accomplished by using a sequence of number or letter patterns displayed on a screen at the speed of one-hundreth of a second. Start with four characters and eventually work your way up to as many as eight characters. Your high performance vision trainer will tally your score based on remembering the characters and their sequence in each pattern.

To increase the level of difficulty, your coach may project the letters or numbers and then instruct you to call out the characters in a particular sequence. For example:

A R X

Z L O

M E B

In this block of letters, your trainer may call out, "Upper left to lower right!" In which case, the answer would be: A, L, B.

Lastly, sport-specific images may be projected at one-hundreth of a second to train speed of recognition. For example, the hand of a pitcher throwing a variety of pitches (e.g., fastball, slider, curveball) may be shown.

EYE CHART WHILE IN MOTION

To train your dynamic acuity, your trainer may utilize a standard eye chart and a mini trampoline or jump rope. With the eye chart set up twenty feet away from you at eye level, you will be asked to jump up and down either on the mini trampoline or by using the jump rope while reading the letters on the chart from top to bottom. Once you've mastered this task, you should attempt to read the letters left to right, right to left, by column, etc.

TURNTABLE WHILE MOVING ON PRO FITTER

This exercise is also geared towards increasing your dynamic acuity. You will need a turntable (see Figure 7.7), letters and numbers arranged from the center to the periphery of a poster board that has been cut to fit this turntable, and a Pro Fitter. While shifting back and forth on the Pro Fitter, you will be asked to call out the letters and numbers from the center to the periphery of a specifically chosen line as fast and as accurately as possible.

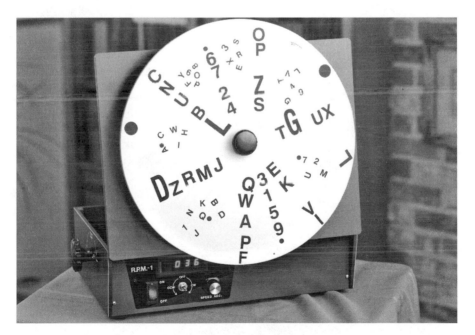

Figure 7.7. Turntable

This motorized turntable rotates a disc with letters and numbers that run from the center to the periphery of the circle and must be identified by the test subject. Speed may be adjusted to increase difficulty.

YOKED PRISM GLASSES

Yoked prism glasses may be used to train visual-motor balancing skill. Light rays that pass through prism lenses get redirected in the opposite direction from the thickest portion of the prism (the base). When prisms are placed before both eyes with the base of each lens on the right side of the eyes (or both on the left side) the result is known as "yoked prisms." These yoked prisms shift the object being viewed in the opposite direction from where it is actually situated, which can be quite unnerving. (See Figure 7.8.)

Try putting a golf ball while wearing these special eyeglasses. In order to succeed, your brain must adjust to the artificial shift in space to achieve the desired result. Try catching a ball while wearing yoked prisms and balancing on a Pro Fitter or some other balancing device—not an easy task! But don't forget that the more extreme the training conditions, the easier the playing field conditions become. Try bunting a Marsden Ball with a special rolling pin while wearing yoked prisms as you balance on a Pro Fitter. Repetitive practice utilizing this equipment will greatly improve your balance on the playing field during intense competition.

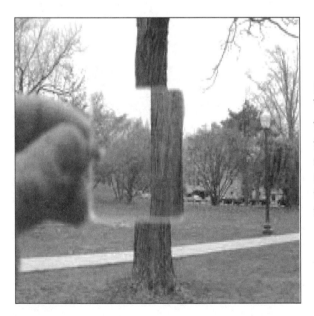

**Figure 7.8.
Yoked Prism Glasses**

These glasses feature lenses that have been designed to shift objects in space to appear displaced from where the test subject would expect them to be.

SLIDE PRESENTATION

To enhance your speed of recognition and visual memory, your trainer may create a slide presentation of a certain sporting activity and project it on a screen or wall. For example, a hockey goalie would be shown a slide presentation of a hockey puck shot on goal from different angles and positions. This hockey goalie would react to these "shot on goal" slides as they are shown at one-hundreth of a second.

Trainers can use slides for any number of sports or playing situations. Skiers may be asked to simulate skiing movements while balancing on a Pro Fitter and viewing slides of flags and moguls in sequence along a ski course. The slides should change rapidly enough to ensure a fluid rhythm on the Pro Fitter, causing the skier to shift back and forth to avoid the obstacles along the terrain. By concentrating and anticipating changes appropriately, the skier should hope to achieve a flawless run. The athlete being trained should aim to view the slides as fast as possible while minimizing errors in movement.

TYPICAL TRAINING PROGRAM

If you opt to enroll in a professionally guided high performance vision training program at a center or clinic, it would be helpful to know what to expect.

A typical weekly session can be anywhere from thirty minutes to an hour in length. In the first of a dozen weeks, emphasis is placed on exercises focused on strengthening proper eye alignment, appreciation of stereo vision, eye tracking, flexibility of focus from near-field to far-field and vice versa, and getting the eyes to work better together as a team. The time is often spent concentrating on five or so exercises in the clinic. This is supplemented by more portable equipment that the athlete takes home each week to work on two to four drills daily in between weekly office sessions. As the sessions progress, the demand placed on the athlete to achieve success becomes more intense. Sometimes the complexity of the drill shifts from one eye at a time to a more challenging two-eyed version of the technique in order to enhance binocular vision.

As mentioned earlier, the first phase of training may be considered visual calisthenics. These exercises have been designed to improve general visual skills before moving on to the second phase of training, which deals with sport-specific visual-cognitive motor issues. Phase one typically lasts five sessions. In phase two (weeks six to ten), the exercises address improving instant visual memory, eye-hand or eye-foot coordination, balance, peripheral awareness, concentration, anticipation, and reaction time. Week eleven is dedicated to teaching the finer points of relaxation, visualization, and positive imagery training, getting the athlete ready to face the competition, secure in the knowledge that his eyes are working at an optimal level. The final week of the clinical program is typically a reassessment of performance scores as they compare to initial results recorded on day one, before the start of training.

CONCLUSION

The purpose of this book is to demonstrate that all of us are capable of greater vision through a better understanding of how the eyes work and how visual skills may be elevated to higher levels than possessed by the average individual. Professionally monitored clinical training offers access to advanced technology and a more systematic path towards gaining a competitive edge. Nevertheless, a home-based program of eye exercises and drills can be extremely effective and should not be discounted. A two-pronged approach, in fact, may be the ideal option. The next chapter looks at a multitude of sport-specific drills that may be done on your own quite easily, whether at home or on the playing field.

8.

Sport-Specific Eye Exercises

ifferent sports demand different skills. As a result, different drills can assure more productive results. This chapter provides a diverse sampling of on-the-field visual-motor exercises that you can practice on a daily basis to hone your sport-specific talents. These simple exercises are challenging, focusing not only on sport-specific skills but also on various components of each sport. As always, the more you practice, the better your results will become.

BASEBALL OR SOFTBALL DRILLS

It has been said that the most difficult and demanding visual skill in sports is the act of hitting a baseball. After all, a player who finds success only three out of every ten times at bat is likely to be considered for the Hall of Fame. But batting prowess does not necessarily result in a golden glove in the field. Therefore, drills are divided to address both the hitting and fielding components of baseball. Understandably, these same exercises apply to softball players as well.

Hitting Drills

Use three baseballs or softballs, each of a different color. One color should signify a bunt, one should signify a full swing, and the last should signify refraining from swinging. As batter, you must react accordingly as soon as you recognize the color of the ball. This drill requires the help of a pitcher, of course.

Another exercise is strobe hitting, in which the batter uses a strobe light or strobe-light glasses while self-tossing balls. The slower the strobe light flashes, the more difficult it is to hit the ball. People at risk of seizure, however, should not use strobe lights to train.

To prepare your eyes for live pitching, color a ball between the inside seams and have someone throw a variety of pitches from the mound. As batter, you should pick up the spin of the ball as quickly as possible, call out the pitch, and watch the ball end its flight in the catcher's mitt. If you are having trouble identifying the pitch, have the pitcher state the pitch before he throws it. This should help you learn to identify types of pitches at their release points. Don't hit the ball during this exercise; just monitor its trajectory.

Another good exercise asks the pitcher to name the area of the field (right, left, or center) to which he would like the ball hit right before he's about to pitch. If the batter hits the ball to the wrong area of the field or pops up, then players switch positions. The pitcher may call for the batter not to swing. If the batter swings on such a call, then players switch roles. The batter may also keep his eyes closed until the pitcher calls, "Open!" If the player swings upon opening his eyes but no ball has been thrown, then players switch positions.

In the release drill, the pitcher simulates a pitch, presenting one to five fingers to the batter instead of actually throwing a ball. The batter is required to call out the number of fingers shown after the pitcher's release. The batter then swings. Next, the batter calls out the number of fingers that a coach, standing six feet in front of the outside corner of the plate, is displaying. This drill teaches the player to pick up the pitch at the release and to keep his head down on the swing. It can be made more difficult by having the pitcher use a ball and show pitches to the hitter without releasing the ball. The hitter would make the visual shift to the plate and hit a sock ball, wiffle ball, or tennis ball off a tee after calling out the pitch.

To make the drill even harder, replace the single tee with a double tee, placing the inside tee (the higher one) about four feet in front of the inside corner of the tee box and the second tee (the lower one) equal to the front point of the outside corner of the tee box. The batter is now forced to see the ball at the release and react to the pitch. If the pitcher shows a fastball, the batter must hit the ball off the inside tee. If the batter reads an off-speed pitch, he must drive the ball to right field off the outside tee. Reverse the tees for left-handed batters.

To add a higher degree of difficulty to these drills, use sock balls (balled up pairs of socks taped up to be smaller than baseballs) or small wiffle balls. In addition, you may use a Thunderstick (see Figure 8.1) training bat, which is much thinner than a regular bat but still feels the same to swing.

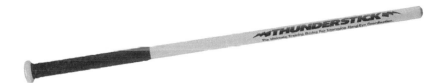

Figure 8.1. Easton Thunderstick Training Bat

This bat is thin but heavily weighted. It is used to train baseball or softball hitters to make contact with the ball under the condition of a limited contact point.

Fielding Drills

As a fielding drill, take five or six balls and number or letter them— one letter or number per ball. Have a trainer hit ground balls. The fielder should call out the letter or number on the ball as he fields it and comes up to throw.

Another drill asks the fielder to close her eyes, open them only after he hears the bat make contact with the ball, and then to catch the grounder or fly ball. The fielder could also lie on his back and stand up as soon as he hears the sound of contact.

In what is called the "shade drill," a runner interferes with the batted ground ball by crossing the path between the ball and the fielder. An outfielder's exercise known as the "fixation drill" is designed to keep the fielder's head steady, demanding that the player run on her toes while fixating on the top of a flagpole or anything stationary and high. The coach then calls out the direction the player should turn or run.

In the "feel drill," the player assumes her position in the field and his coach delivers grounders or fly balls. After retrieving the ball, the player closes his eyes as he is about to throw the ball to a predetermined location. This same drill may be used with pitchers to develop better control.

Concentration Technique

How many times has your coach urged you to keep your eye on the ball? These words of encouragement have always bothered me. Coaches may know how to teach proper batting technique, but when it comes to teaching their players how to keep their eyes on the ball, most of them haven't a clue. There is, in fact, a step-by-step approach to learning this skill.

Like all aspects of the game of baseball, these skills should be practiced year round, both on and off of the field. As the game begins, the batter should identify the pitcher's type of release (e.g., over-the-top, three-quarter, side-arm). The on-deck circle then becomes the stage for the batter to come, who should visualize and even vocalize positive thoughts such as, "I love to hit on this field. I own this pitcher."

When the batter is in the box, he needs to clear her mind and concentrate on seeing the ball. For example, this may be achieved by seeing, in the mind's eye, the letter "R" in the Rawlings logo on the baseball. This ritual eliminates the distractions batters bring to the plate and focuses attention on the job at hand, which is to see the ball and hit it.

TENNIS DRILLS

Take a standard tennis ball and put four circles of the same color on different parts of the ball. Do this with a number of balls and use different colors. The player should then call out the color of the ball coming at her at any time before it makes contact with her racquet. This teaches the player to follow the ball all the way to the racquet. To increase the level of difficulty, make the colored circles smaller and smaller.

To study rotation, use a standard two-colored ball when rallying and serving. The goal is to identify the spin, call it out, and react appropriately. Increase the speed to make the task harder.

To enhance your ability to identify a serve, have your trainer show you the two types of serves to name. Your coach would then

---

As the pitcher sets up to throw, the batter should soft focus on the pitcher's cap (for an over-the-top release), face (for a three-quarter release), or chest (for a side-arm pitch).

As the pitcher separates his hands to throw to the plate, the batter should make a horizontal shift of his eyes to the release point of the ball and pick up the type of pitch about to arrive. The batter is now fine centering (intense focus) on the process of tracking the ball to his bat. Remember, this is much more effective if the batter attempts to look for the letter "R" in Rawlings on the baseball rather than just at the baseball. (Note: It is extremely rare for a batter to see this letter "R" all the way to the bat. That is really not important. What is important is that he *believes* he is tracking the letter "R" all the way to the bat. This will make him a far better hitter.)

It goes without saying that if the batter believes the pitch will be a ball and chooses not to swing, he must still track the letter R on the baseball all the way to the catcher's glove. This will reinforce the batter's ability to keep his eye on the ball. Effort made on a regular basis reinforces muscle memory.

---

attempt to serve and you would identify the serve as quickly as possible. This exercise teaches players to look at the contact point of the serve and be able to identify and react to the speed, location, and type of serve offered. Have your coach add more types of serves as you get better at this task.

To improve reaction time, keep your eyes closed until you hear the ball contact your opponent's racquet, and then try to locate the ball and return the volley. Instead of closing your eyes, you could also turn your back to the server instead and wait to react to the sound of the ball hitting the racquet. You could also lie on your back and pop up when you hear the sound of the ball being hit.

In the strobe serve drill, the player practices his serve on the court while wearing strobe-light glasses. The goal is to enhance the player's concentration through visual noise. Slowing the strobe light increases the difficulty level.

Finally, you could use two balls of different colors and react differently to each ball. For example, if the ball served is green, then you are required to lob it back. This drill forces the player to think and react on his feet. Add a different colored ball and more commands to make the exercise a little harder to accomplish.

GOLF DRILLS

Localization, fixation, and perception result from complex interactions between the object being viewed, the structures of the eye, and the brain. Alignment of a putter, a golf ball, and a hole on the green involve these complicated functions combined with variations in refractive error (your eyeglasses prescription) and peripheral viewing phenomena.

An individual's keenest eyesight occurs when viewing objects directly and utilizing central, or foveal, vision. Putt alignment, however, requires both downward and lateral gazes (possibly combined with elevation or depression of gaze on greens that are not level from the point of lie). The player, therefore, must employ peripheral fixation to determine alignment. Humans interpret position and distance of an object (in this case, the hole) utilizing various monocular and binocular clues to depth. The greater the distance, the less we depend on binocular (two-eye) clues. Shadow, texture, and contour contribute to the awareness of distance and position. We all interpret these clues slightly differently. The final computation in the brain encompasses interpretations of retinal stimuli from both eyes. Since the peripheral retina is less sensitive than the central retina, precise accuracy suffers. Under ideal circumstances, without wearing glasses, the average golfer has a problem. Add nearsightedness, farsightedness, or astigmatism and the problem is compounded. The prescription of a pair of glasses is truly only accurate in the center of the lens. When we view objects off to the side, there is a distortion due to prismatic effect, making alignment a little bit more difficult.

According to one study, 80 percent of golfers aligned their putters outside of one inch from the center of the hole from a distance of only four feet. A full 50 percent of golfers failed to align within approximately two inches of the center of the hole. These golfers were actually aligned poorly enough to miss the hole. This phenomenon is a common visual occurrence, as, in actuality, golfers typify the average person. Few of us possess the unusual acuity and spatial awareness of a naval aviator. The ability to perceive minuscule spatial separations occurs rarely. In other words, the average individual functions with slightly less sensitive neurological connections, and slightly less precise brain processing to localize and align objects. Although this situation may be called an inborn error of development, it may be classified as a normal variation of the human visual mechanism.

The fact is that the average athlete's performance suffers as a result of the normal complexities of the visual system. Quite appropriately, most people could probably improve performance by utilizing a laser sight on the putter to compensate for the subtle but normal inaccuracies of the eyes. There is a variety of training drills, however, that can help you noticeably improve your golf score without resorting to cheating.

To work on putting alignment, place the ball at your feet with the logo positioned on an imaginary straight line aimed at the cup. Visualize a path or trough traveling from the head of your club to the cup. Position your dominant eye directly over the ball and putt.

To improve your distance prediction, visualize how many heel-to-toe steps you will need to reach the cup from any random position on the green, and then walk the distance to test your estimate.

The plumb bobbing exercise is an effective way to recognize subtle breaks in the green. Stand eight to ten feet behind the ball. While in a crouching position (like a baseball catcher's stance), hold your putter so that the blade is aimed straight at the hole. Line up the ball and the flagstick with your dominant eye. Be sure to hold the club as straight as possible to ensure a correct read. Make a note of which side of the putting blade the hole appears. If the ball is on the right side of your putter, play a break to the right. If it's on the left side, then play it to the left.

The coin drill may be done on a carpet at home. Place a dime at a chosen putting distance. Place three pennies behind the dime so that they form a triangle. Attempt to putt the ball over the dime and into the pocket created by the three pennies.

BASKETBALL DRILLS

In the ball toss drill, the receiver looks at the passer's eyes and attempts to catch the ball on the fingertips of her extended hands. In the dribble and tennis ball toss drill, the player attempts to catch a tennis ball thrown by a teammate while dribbling a basketball with one hand. Hands should be switched after a period of time.

An important drill is foul shot visualization. While on the foul line, take a few bounces and then set up the basketball with the brand's logo facing you. For example, if the logo is Spalding, focus on the letter "S" in Spalding. Visualize a stream of air carrying this letter just over the front rim of the basket.

Lastly, to perform the chair dribbling drill, set up five chairs spaced about two feet apart in a straight vertical line. Have a teammate stand at each end of the line of chairs facing you. While looking into your teammate's eyes, attempt to weave through the line of chairs while dribbling until you reach the end of the line, and then weave back towards your other teammate at the other end.

SKIING DRILLS

The concentration and anticipation technique is an outstanding drill to reinforce central focus and anticipate changes in terrain while traversing a ski slope. You will need strobe-light glasses and a balance board of some kind. You may purchase a balance board or build one yourself. (See instructions on page 105.) While balanced on the balance board, view a series of slides of flags and moguls in sequence along a ski course. Change the slides rapidly enough to assure a fluid rhythm on the board as you move back and forth trying to avoid the obstacles as they appear.

To continue to improve in this task, increase the speed of the slides while minimizing errors in movement. In addition, the flashing effect of the strobe-light glasses may be made slower to raise the level of difficulty.

Another skiing exercise is the arrows and balance board drill, as mentioned in Chapter 6. (See page 106.) Take a poster board and draw sixteen bold arrows on it. Attach the board to a wall at eye level about eight feet away or farther. While on the balance board, shift your weight in concert with the direction of the arrows left to right. Time yourself to see how fast you can accomplish all the shifts indicated by the arrows. Rotate the poster board one turn and start again. The goal is to improve your reaction time.

FOOTBALL DRILLS

To improve the eye-hand coordination of a wide receiver, tight end, running back, or defensive secondary player, a coach may stand behind the player as he faces a wall from about three feet away and proceed to toss tennis balls with large permanent marker numbers written on them at the wall. The player should attempt to catch each ball, calling out its number as he watches it come into his hands. The athlete should strive to keep her head as steady as possible, letting his eyes do all the work in tracking the ball coming off the wall.

Another great training exercise involves a computer slide presentation depicting different pictures of offensive and defensive formations from a quarterback's perspective. These play formations are projected onto a large screen at a very rapid exposure speed (perhaps one-hundreth of a second). The quarterback is asked to reveal the offensive and defensive formations observed as accurately as possible.

The Zone

We've all heard great athletes extol the virtues of being "in the zone," but what is the "zone" and how do you get in it? To better understand this concept, consider athletes who have been in the zone. They report being hyper-aware of their environments, seeing things more clearly, interpreting movements in slow motion, not thinking about their bodies or athletic techniques, and feeling relaxed and stress-free.

To enter the zone, brainwaves must achieve "alpha state," which is a heightened level of mental suggestibility that enhances relaxation and concentration. How can you achieve alpha state? First, try progressive relaxation. Be seated with your legs uncrossed or lie down. Wear ear plugs or listen to soft music through headphones to eliminate outside noise. Proceed to tense your facial muscles for three seconds, keep these muscles fixed as such for another three seconds, and then release them and relax for three seconds. Follow this action by performing the same ritual with your fists, biceps, chest, abdomen, buttocks, thighs, calves, feet, and toes.

Take five deep breaths, starting with an inhalation from your diaphragm and working your way up to your nose. Then exhale

HOCKEY DRILLS

Hockey is a very fast-moving game. Quick decisions are critical to scoring or preventing a goal. A variety of drills can raise the threshold of quickness for skaters and goaltenders alike. You can purchase a variable-speed strobe light and set the flash to pulsate at a relatively slow speed while in a dark room. The task at hand for a goalie would be to stop shots on goal while enduring these brief moments of light and dark. Similarly, skaters can practice scoring goals or passing while dealing with the same difficulties associated with such an environment. Always remember, of course, that studies have shown that individuals who suffer from epileptic seizures

---

through your mouth with the breath working its way back down towards your diaphragm. Think of this breathing technique as filling up a glass of water from the bottom up and then emptying it from the top to the bottom.

Next, visualize yourself slowly walking down a flight of ten stairs. With each step, silently verbalize an adjective that represents relaxation to you. Tell yourself that each step will make you feel increasingly calm and relaxed. Finally, picture yourself at a real or imaginary place of amazing tranquility. It could be a private beach, a row boat in the middle of a quiet lake, or whatever works for you. The more vivid your visualizations are, the better the results will be.

Now, in your alpha state, see yourself succeeding. Be specific. Visualize your mechanics from every viewpoint (front, back, and both sides). See positives only. Count slowly from one to five. With each number, reinforce how great and relaxed you feel. At the count of five, tell yourself that you will feel the best you have felt in a long time upon opening your eyes, that you are ready to go for the gold.

Experts contend that any athlete can train to be in the zone. The technical term is "cybernetics," or programming yourself for success through visualization. Your body will learn what to do if you learn how to tell it what to do properly.

should avoid practicing this type of drill, as the stroboscopic effect has been shown to trigger seizures on occasion in this population.

Another great drill for a goaltender is to have a skater shoot pucks of different colors at the net. He must call out the color of each puck as he attempts to stop the shot. To vary this drill, put a large number on each puck for the goalie to identify. Even if it is almost impossible for the goalie to identify the number during the exercise, the effort he makes to discern the number on the puck will train him to track the puck into his glove or stick for a longer duration. Finally, rapid projected images of shots on goal may be used by a goalie to train reaction accuracy and speed.

CONCLUSION

It is safe to say that there is no shortage of visual-cognitive motor exercises that may be used to meet the numerous demands of almost any type of sport. The only limit is your own imagination. While different sports place specific visual demands on athletes, and thus require athletes to perform particular exercises to train optimally, many of the drills described in this chapter may be easily adapted to meet the needs of a plethora of sports. Overall, an athlete can only get better if he seeks to improve his eye-hand (and eye-foot) coordination, tracking and flexibility of focus, concentration, timing, and anticipation, all of which may benefit from a number of different eye exercises.

9.

Putting It All Together

If you are an athlete and you've been to an eyecare professional, you can probably recall that efforts were made by the doctor to confirm that the external and internal structures of your eyes were healthy and to improve your visual acuity. Without a doubt, these two aspects of the eyecare field are of paramount importance to the status of your vision. It is important for eye doctors to measure basic visual abilities and attempt to compensate for any visual deficits with such measures as eyeglasses, contact lenses, or corrective surgical procedures. The intention of high performance vision, however, is to reveal that there is more that may be done when it comes to vision and athletic excellence.

What are your overall goals in reference to your vision and your chosen sport? What did you hope to gain by reading this book? Was it to find that elusive competitive edge that all athletes crave? What is it about your vision and your sport that demands careful attention? What problems have you been experiencing in your game that may be directly or indirectly related to your eyes?

To understand the role vision plays in your athletic activities, you must first learn about the components of the incredible organ known as the human eye. By familiarizing yourself with the functions of the many parts of the ocular system, you will recognize the fact that these functions may be trained and maximized to give you better vision than you ever thought possible. You don't have to settle at merely healthy eyes and adequate eyesight. You can achieve high performance vision.

Vision plays the most significant role in athletic competition. Thankfully, eye training may be accomplished in a variety of ways. There is a wealth of drills and techniques that may be performed at home or on the playing field to get you on your way to success. For those athletes who seek a more monitored approach to gaining a competitive edge, the newest and most sophisticated eye-training technology may be found in the rapidly growing number of clinics offering visual-cognitive motor training, and high performance vision specialists are becoming more and more common.

There are also sport-specific drills and exercises that can benefit you in your chosen activity. Sports, of course, come with the potential for injury, so it is crucial to know the details of the most common eye injuries and how these problems may be prevented.

As much as this book attempts to leave no stone unturned, for every question answered, another one may have popped up in its place. Consider this a good thing. More questions simply mean you are moving in the right direction on your course to visual excellence and success in your game. *High Performance Vision* is the primer to get you on your way. Don't forget to enjoy the journey!

Conclusion

I am confident that this book has confirmed your appreciation of the major role your eyes play not only in sports but in life in general. These pages were designed to change the way you approach your eyes and entire visual system, and to shed light on the power of high performance vision training. As is the case with so much of what we do in our daily routines, of course, practice makes perfect. Repetition and ongoing training is the secret to maintaining a competitive edge. Hopefully, when you hear the term "muscle memory" from now on, you will realize that so much of muscle memory is driven by the sensory system, of which vision is a huge part.

Maintaining a regimen of these eye exercises for twenty minutes twice a week will keep your visual system in shape. As they say, "Practice! Practice! Practice!" If repetitive practice were of no value, then why would elite ball players take batting practice before every baseball or softball game? Why would golfers take hundreds of putts on the putting green as part of their training regimens? Why would basketball players take so many shots from the free throw line between games? Nevertheless, you don't have to embrace this program on my word alone. Try it and truly see.

Resources

While doctors in the field of high performance vision training are becoming more and more common, there are a handful of professionals who have the expertise to suit your needs right now. If you are looking to improve your vision and live in any one of the designated states, the following specialists may be consulted. In addition, should you decide to train at home, this section contains a number of companies from which you can purchase the necessary equipment to hone your eyesight and achieve athletic excellence.

HIGH PERFORMANCE VISION DOCTORS

ALABAMA

Dr. Mark Schaeffer
Schaeffer Eye Center
3431 Colonnade Parkway
Birmingham, AL 35243
(205) 967-2020
drmschaeffer@schaeffereyecenter
  .com
www.schaeffereyecenter.com

CALIFORNIA

Dr. Bronson Hamada
Surf City Optometry (Visual
  Speed Inc.)
7192 Edinger Avenue
Huntington Beach, CA 92647
(714) 848-1400
TheOC@SurfCityOptometry.com
www.SurfCityOptometry.com

COLORADO

**Dr. H. Jeff Ward, F.I.A.O.,
  Diplomate of the American
  Board of Optometry**
Highlands Ranch Optical / The
  Rocky Mountain Sports Vision
  Institute
9370 S. Colorado Boulevard,
  Suite A4
Highlands Ranch, CO 80126
(720) 344-2020
hjeffward@comcast.net
www.highlandsranchoptical.com

CONNECTICUT

Dr. Jennifer Stewart
Norwalk Eye Care
5 Eversley Avenue
Norwalk, CT 06851
(203) 853-1010
JstewartOD@yahoo.com
www.norwalkeyecare.com

FLORIDA

Dr. Robert Davis
Dr. Amanda Nanasy
The Eye Center
1732 University Drive
Pembroke Pines, FL 33024
(954) 432-7711
eyesail@mindspring.com
www.eyecenter.com

Dr. Carl Spear
Dr. Katie Gilbert-Spear
Dr. Mark Obenchain
Robert Constantine, OTR/L
The Visual Performance Center
5101 North Davis Highway
Pensacola, FL 32503
(850) 479-7379
chspear@gmail.com
www.vpcpensacola.com

Dr. Don Teig
Executive Director, "The A Team,
  High Performance Vision
  Associates"
Ultimate Events, LLC
3111 North Ocean Drive, Suite 1212
Hollywood, FL 33019
(203) 312-3123
don@ultimateeventsllc.com
www.ultimateeventsllc.com
www.highperformancevision
  associates.com

INDIANA

Dr. Jeremy Ciano
RevolutionEYES
14250 Clay Terrace Boulevard,
  Suite 160
Carmel, IN 46032
(317) 844-2020
DrCiano@Revolution-EYES.com
www.Revolution-EYES.com

Dr. Rajender Macha
Peak Visual Performance
1607 South Scatterfield Road
Anderson, IN 46016
(765) 649-1200
peakvisualperformance.net

Dr. Charles Shearer
Center for Eyecare Excellence
517 Lincolnway East
Mishawaka, IN 46544
(574) 255-1231
Bernellconsult@aol.com
www.eyesongrace.com
www.bernell.com

IOWA

Dr. DeAnn Fitzgerald
Dr. Kathy Hotsenpiller
Dr. D.M. Fitzgerald & Associates
3225 Williams Parkway SW, Suite 1
Cedar Rapids, IA 52404
(319) 366-3500
docfitzgerald.eyecare@gmail.com
www.docfitzgerald.com

KANSAS

Dr. Aaron Wilmes
Lawrence Optometric Center
930 Iowa Street, Suite 3
Lawrence, KS 66044
(785) 842-1242
arwilmes@LawrenceOptometric
  Center.com
www.lawrenceoptometriccenter
  .com

MASSACHUSETTS

Dr. Robert A. Buonfiglio
Gary G. Kalloch, RDO
Eye on Performance Sports Vision
  Training
11 Cabot Road
Woburn, MA 01801
(781) 231-1100
info@eyeonperformance.net
www.eyeonperformance.net

NEW HAMPSHIRE

Dr. Scott Krauchunas
InFocus Eyecare, Inc
320 Daniel Webster Highway
Belmont, NH 03220
(603) 527-2035
drkrunch@infocuseyecarenh.com
athelite@infocuseyecarenh.com
www.infocuseyecarenh.com

NEW YORK

Dr. Fred Edmunds
XTREMESIGHT Performance
274 West Main Street
Victor, NY 14564
(585) 880-4818
drfred@xtremesight.com
www.xtremesightperformance.com

NORTH CAROLINA

Dr. Charlene Henderson
Dr. Tracy MacIntyre Raykovicz
Sports Vision Carolina at Blink
  Eye Care
16618 Riverstone Way
Charlotte, NC 28277
(704) 817-3800
sportsvisioncarolina@blinkcharlott
  e.com
www.blinkcharlotte.com

NORTH DAKOTA

Dr. David Biberdorf
Valley Vision Clinic, Ltd. / Valley
  Sports Vision
2200 South Washington Street
Grand Forks, ND 58201
(701) 775-3135
drbiberdorf@valleyvision.net
www.valleyvision.net
www.valleysportsvision.com

TENNESSEE

Dr. Peter Van Hoven
Dr. Ken Young
Dr. Nick Engle
Primary Eye Care Group of
  Middle Tennessee, Brentwood
  Office
205 Ward Circle
Brentwood, TN 37027
(615) 373-0080
PvanHoven@primaryeyecare.com
kyoung@primaryeyecare.com
nengle@primaryeyecare.com
www.pecgbrentwood.com

HIGH PERFORMANCE VISION EQUIPMENT

Bernell Corporation
Mishawaka, IN
(800) 348-2225
www.bernell.com
*Bernell has the largest line of visual
rehabilitation products worldwide and
carries over 2,000 ophthalmic
products.*

DynaVision
8800 Global Way
West Chester, OH 45069
(513) 645-2510
www.dynavisioninternational.com
*Since 1989, Dynavision has
manufactured high-quality
rehabilitation and sports
training devices.*

J.W. Engineering
8 Dike Driver
Wesley Hills, NY 10952
(845) 354-8025
www.jtac.com
J.W. Engineering designs specialized machines for visual rehabilitation.

Lafayette Instrument Company
3700 Sagamore Parkway North
Lafayette, IN 47904
(800) 428-7545
www.lafayetteinstrument.com
Lafayette Instrument is a manufacturer and provider of industry-specific products.

Neurotracker/CogniSens Athletics
5186 Chemin de la Côte-des-Neiges, Suite 4
Montreal, Canada
(855) 480-0808 ext 710
www.cognisensathletics.com (science and sports)
www.neurotracker.net (team and individual sport athletes)
CogniSens Athletics develops technology that measures neurobiological activity in sports.

Sanet Vision
6788 South Kings Ranch Road, Suite 4
Gold Canyon, AZ 85118
(800) 346-4925
www.svivision.com

Sanet Vision manufactures the Sanet Vision Integrator, which contains multiple functions used to measure information processing, visual reaction time, and other neurobiological processes.

Senaptec LLC
2331 NW Jessamine Way
Portland, OR 97229
(888) 855-2091
www.senaptec.com
Senaptec supplies technology that analyzes and improves vision and sensory-motor skills.

SMI SensoMotoric Instruments, Inc.
28 Atlantic Avenue
Boston, MA 02110
(617) 557-0010
www.smivision.com
SMI provides medical solutions, including eye-tracking systems and computer vision applications.

SVT Sports Vision Trainer
58 Park Road
Burwood, Sydney, Australia
612 9747-2518
www.sportsvision.com.au
The SVT Sports Vision Trainer helps sharpen visual-motor reaction time and improve hand-eye coordination in both athletes and non-athletes.

ULTIMEYES
Carrot Neurotechnology, Inc.
23679 Calabasas Road, Suite 796
Calabasas, CA 91302
(818) 796-3842
www.ultimeyesvision.com

Ultimeyes is a mobile application available for purchase, designed to train the user's eyes to improve vision and visual processing.

Vision Coach
6380 Rancho Park Drive
San Diego, CA 92120
(877) 826-2240
www.visioncoachtrainer.com

The Vision Coach, invented by Robin Donley, is an interactive light board used for visual rehabilitation.

Wayne Engineering
8242 North Christiana Avenue
Skokie, IL 60076
(847) 674-7166
www.wayneengineering.com

Wayne Engineering develops machines for optometry and sports vision training.

About the Author

Dr. Donald S. Teig, OD, FAAO, received his BA in psychology from the University of Buffalo and his BS and OD from the Pennsylvania College of Optometry. He has served as vision consultant to many professional sports teams in areas including baseball, football, and hockey. As past president of the International Academy of Sports Vision, prior chairman of the Sports Vision Section of the American Optometric Association, and former director of the Institute for Sports Vision in Ridgefield, Connecticut, Dr. Teig works with a multidisciplinary network of sports medicine experts.

Beginning over forty years ago, Dr. Teig pioneered work in sports vision and visual-motor performance training with major league baseball. Subsequently, Dr. Teig and his associates have worked with over fifteen major league baseball clubs, pro golf and tennis tours, several NBA basketball clubs, many Olympic teams, professional football and hockey teams, and dancers of the Joffrey Ballet.

Dr. Teig has written numerous articles on the relationship of vision to improved athletic performance. He has lectured throughout the world on this topic, and has developed much of the equipment and techniques being used in the field today. As a sports-vision specialist, Dr. Teig has appeared on several network television and radio programs, including featured segments of *The Today Show, Dateline NBC, ESPN Sports Center, The View,* and programs on HBO. He has also contributed to sports segments on New York's all-sports radio station, WFAN, earning him the nickname "Doctor Jock."

147

Permissions

Figure 2.1 courtesy of Blausen.com staff. "Blausen gallery 2014." Wikiversity Journal of Medicine. DOI:10.15347/wjm/2014.010. ISSN 20018762.

Figures 4.1, 4.2, 4.4, 4.5, 4.7, 4.10, 4.19, 6.1, 6.3, 6.4, 6.6, 6.7, 7.5, 7.6, and 7.8 reproduced with permission from Bernell, a Division of Vision Training Products, Inc.

Figures 4.3 and 4.9 courtesy of Lafayette Instrument Company, Inc.

Figures 4.8, 4.11, 4.12, 4.15, 4.17, 6.2, 6.11, 6.12, and 8.1 courtesy of Donald Teig.

Figure 4.13 courtesy of Joe Ward/The New York Times; illustrations by Carol Fabricatore.

Figure 4.14 courtesy of Carl Zeiss Meditec Inc.

Figure 4.16 courtesy of Wikimedia Commons, the free media repository. User: Jeff Dahl.

Figure 4.18 courtesy of Perform Better.

Figures 4.6 and 6.9 courtesy of Jayson Teig, Image Is Everything.

Figure 6.8 courtesy of ULTIMEYES by Carrot Neurotechnology, Inc.

Figure 6.10 courtesy of The Quick Board, Memphis, TN.

Figure 7.1 courtesy of SensoMotoric Instruments (SMI).

Figures 7.2 and 7.3 courtesy of NeuroTracker.net. Your path to improvement.

Figure 7.4 used by permission, King-Devick Test, Inc 2015.

Figure 7.7 courtesy of J.W. Engineering.

Index

Accommodation, 59, 61, 82,
    89–91, 112
Accommodative flippers, 112
Aging vision. *See* Presbyopia.
Alignment, 44–45, 83, 96
Allergies, 30–31
Anterior chamber, 16, 34
Anticipation timing, 45–46, 82,
    103
Aqueous humor, 15

Balance board, 75–77, 94,
    105–106, 133
Baseball
    drills, 125–128
    hitting a, 62–65
Basketball drills, 132
Basketball, protective eyewear,
    38
Bassin Anticipation Timer
    (B.A.T.), 46–47, 103
B.A.T. *See* Bassin Anticipation
    Timer.
Bernell corporation, 89–90
Beta-carotene, 67
Billy Board, 75–76
Blepharitis, 30

Blowout fracture. *See* Orbital
    trauma.
Brock String technique, 56–57
Bull's-Eye Card, 99

Carotenoids, 66
Cataract, 21, 30, 40
Cliradex, 30
Color vision, 46, 48–49
Concentration technique, 109,
    128–129
Cones, 16–17, 46, 66
Conjunctiva, 32
Conjunctivitis (Pink eye), 30–31
Contact lenses, 18, 23, 30, 33
    astigmatism, 25
    contrast sensitivity, 23
    convenience, 24
    ease of handling, 24
    no-feel comfort, 24
    optic zones and oversized
        diameters, 25
    stability and durability, 24
    uncompromising to corneal
        health, 24
    water content, 25

151

Contrast sensitivity, 49, 82–83, 100
Convergence, building, 96–97
Cornea, 16, 26–27, 32–33
Corneal abrasion, 33
Corneal molding, 18, 25–26
Corneal refractive therapy. *See* Corneal molding.
Correcting vision, 18
CSV-1000, 49–50
Cycloplegia drop, 33–34

Demodex, 30
Depth perception, 50–52, 55, 57, 74, 83–84, 102–103, 119
Detached retina, 33–34, 38
Developmental Eye Movement test, 117
Diplopia. *See* Double vision.
Divergence, building, 96
Doctor, high performance vision, 13
Dominant eye, 52–54, 95–96, 106, 112, 132
Double vision, 35–36
Dry eye, 26–27, 31–32
Dynamic visual acuity, 74, 83, 120–121

Easton Thunderstick training bat, 127
Esophoria, 45
Exophoria, 45
Eye
 anatomy of, 15–17
 conditions, 29–32. *See also* Blepharitis; Cataract; Conjunctivitis (Pink eye); Dry   eye; Pinguecula and pterygium.

injuries, 33–38. *See also* Corneal abrasion; Detached retina; Hyphema; Impaired vision from concussion or head trauma; Lid laceration; Orbital trauma (Blowout fracture); Ruptured or lacerated globe.
Eyeglasses, 18–23
Eye-hand-foot coordination, 54–55
Eye-movement skill, 55–56
Eye teaming, 56–57, 84, 97--99
Eye-to-foot speed and patterning, 57, 84, 104
Eye-to-hand speed, 61, 84–85
Eye-to-hand-to-foot-to-body coordination, 84, 106–107, 119
Eyewear, protective, 38–40
 basketball, 38
 football, 40
 hockey, 40
 racquet sports, 39
 skiing, 39
 swimming and water sports, 39

Far-sightedness. *See* Hyperopia.
Field analyzers, 67–68
First aid kit for ocular emergencies, 37
Flashlight tag, 92
Focus flexibility, 59, 61, 82, 89–91
Focusing Flippers, 60–61
Football
 drills, 133–134
 protective eyewear, 40
Fovea, 16

Vision Coach, 71
Visual adjustability, 74
Visual concentration, 74, 86
Visual cortex, 16
Visual-motor balancing skills, 75, 86–87, 122
Visual Motor Enhancement System (VMET), 54–55, 117–118
Visual skills, measuring. *See* Measuring visual skills.
Visual tracings, 90–91
Visualization, 77
Vitamin A, 67
Vitreous humor, 16, 34
VLT. *See* Visible light transmission.

VMET. *See* Visual Motor Enhancement System.

Wayne Accommodative Focusing Device, 59, 61
Wayne Balance Board, 76–77
Wayne PAT. *See* Wayne Peripheral Awareness Trainer.
Wayne Peripheral Awareness Trainer, 119–120
Wayne Saccadic Fixator, 55, 77, 117–118

Yoked prism glasses, 122

Zeaxanthin, 41, 66

WHAT YOU MUST KNOW ABOUT FOOD AND SUPPLEMENTS FOR OPTIMAL VISION CARE
Ocular Nutrition Handbook

Jeffrey Anshel, OD

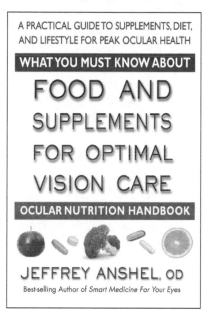

As children, we were told to eat our carrots if we wanted good eyesight. Carrots contain beta-carotene, which the body can convert into vitamin A— a necessary nutrient for optimal vision. For most of us, that's were our knowledge of vitamins and eye health stops. Over the last twenty years, many studies have demonstrated that certain foods and natural supplements can play a major role in the treatment of eye problems. From the best-selling author of *Smart Medicine for Your Eyes* comes a new, concise guide to these powerful substances.

What You Must Know About Food and Supplements for Optimal Vision Care is divided into three parts. Part One is an overview of nutritional principles. This section explores the function of nutrients that benefit not only the visual system but also the entire body. Part Two provides a list of common eye disorders and includes a brief discussion of each condition, supplying handy charts that detail the nutritional, herbal, and homeopathic treatments that may be used to alleviate each disorder. Part Three offers further guidance by presenting dietary approaches to eye health and providing important information on the interaction of various foods and medications.

By eating mindfully and choosing supplements wisely, there is much you can do to support eye health. In this helpful and easy-to-use resource, Dr. Anshel provides you with a wealth of information on the most effective natural products and foods available to promote optimal vision.

$16.95 US • 176 pages • 6 x 9-inch quality paperback • ISBN 978-0-7570-0410-0

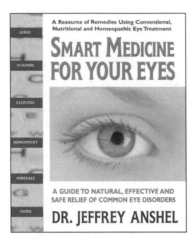

A Resource of Remedies Using Conventional, Nutritional and Homeopathic Eye Treatment

HERBS
VITAMINS
EXERCISES
HOMEOPATHY
MINERALS
FOODS

SMART MEDICINE
FOR YOUR EYES

A GUIDE TO NATURAL, EFFECTIVE AND
SAFE RELIEF OF COMMON EYE DISORDERS

DR. JEFFREY ANSHEL

SMART MEDICINE FOR YOUR EYES
A Guide to Natural, Effective, and Safe Relief of Common Eye Disorders
Jeffrey Anshel, OD

While visiting an eye-care professional is essential, to make informed decisions, you need to understand what's going on with your eyes. That's why *Smart Medicine for Your Eyes* was written. Here is an A-to-Z guide to the most common eye disorders and their treatments, using both conventional and alternative care. This unique book has been carefully designed to give you quick and easy access to up-to-date information and advice regarding your eye's health and function. Part One provides a simple overview of how the eyes work, describes the development of vision, and presents the basic history, theories, and practices of nutritional care, herbal therapy, and homeopathy.

Part Two contains a comprehensive A-to-Z listing of the various eye disorders affecting children and adults, from nearsightedness to styes, from glaucoma to macular degeneration. Each entry clearly explains the problem and offers specific advice using a variety of approaches. Part Two also provides a troubleshooting guide that offers possible causes of common eye symptoms, a first-aid guide for eye and contact-lens emergencies, and a comprehensive table detailing ocular side effects that may be caused by today's most popular systemic medications.

Rounding out the book is Part Three, which presents step-by-step guidance on the specific techniques and procedures suggested in Part Two, including acupressure and acupuncture, eyeglasses and contact lenses, orthokeratolgy and refractive surgery, and vision therapy. Lists of recommended suppliers and resource organizations will help you put the recommendations into practice.

A vital bridge between mainstream medicine and proven traditional therapies, *Smart Medicine for Your Eyes* is a reliable source of information that you will turn to time and time again to protect the greatest of your possessions—your eyes.

$19.95 US • 424 pages • 7.5 x 9-inch quality paperback • ISBN 978-0-7570-0301-1

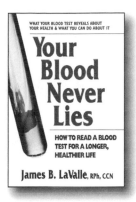

YOUR BLOOD NEVER LIES

How to Read a Blood Test for a Longer, Healthier Life

James B. LaValle, RPh, CCN

A standard blood test indicates how well the kidneys and liver are functioning, the potential for heart disease, and a host of other vital health markers. Unfortunately, most of us cannot decipher these results ourselves or even formulate the right questions to ask about them—or we couldn't, until now.

In *Your Blood Never Lies,* best-selling author James LaValle clears the mystery surrounding blood test results. In simple language, he explains all of the information found on these forms, making it understandable and accessible. This means that you can look at the results yourself and know the significance of each marker. Dr. LaValle even recommends the most effective treatments—both conventional and complementary—for dealing with any problematic findings. Rounding out the book are the names of test markers that should be requested for a more complete physical picture.

A blood test can reveal so much about your body, but only if you can interpret the results. *Your Blood Never Lies* provides the up-to-date information you need to take control of your health.

$16.95 US • 368 pages • 6 x 9-inch quality paperback • ISBN 978-0-7570-0350-9

WHAT YOU MUST KNOW ABOUT VITAMINS, MINERALS, HERBS & MORE

Choosing the Nutrients That Are Right for You

Pamela Wartian Smith, MD, MPH

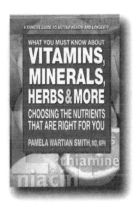

What You Must Know About Vitamins, Minerals, Herbs & More guides you in restoring and maintaining health through the wise use of nutrients. Part One discusses the individual nutrients necessary for well-being, Part Two offers nutritional programs for a wide variety of health concerns, and Part Three presents supplementation plans. Whether you want to preserve good health or overcome a medical condition, this book will give you the information you need to make the best nutritional choices possible.

$15.95 US • 448 pages • 6 x 9-inch quality paperback • ISBN 978-0-7570-0233-5

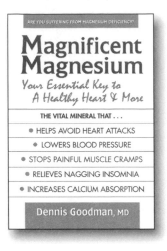

ARE YOU SUFFERING FROM MAGNESIUM DEFICIENCY?

Magnificent Magnesium

Your Essential Key to A Healthy Heart & More

THE VITAL MINERAL THAT . . .

• HELPS AVOID HEART ATTACKS

• LOWERS BLOOD PRESSURE

• STOPS PAINFUL MUSCLE CRAMPS

• RELIEVES NAGGING INSOMNIA

• INCREASES CALCIUM ABSORPTION

Dennis Goodman, MD

MAGNIFICENT MAGNESIUM

Your Essential Key to a Healthy Heart & More

Dennis Goodman, MD

Despite the development of many "breakthrough" drugs designed to combat its effects, heart disease remains the number-one killer of Americans. Is there a simpler solution? The answer is yes. For many years, scientists and medical researchers have known about a common mineral that can effectively prevent or remedy many cardiovascular conditions. And unlike the pharmaceuticals usually prescribed, this supplement has no dangerous side effects. In this book, world-renowned cardiologist Dr. Dennis Goodman shines a spotlight on magnesium, the mineral that can maximize your heart health.

The author first establishes a firm foundation for understanding heart disease, detailing its many forms and providing a brief overview of its fundamental mechanisms. Next, he examines the important role magnesium plays in many life processes and explores how a deficiency of this substance can lead to many of our nation's most common health conditions, including cardiovascular disease. The author then details magnesium's astounding benefits, not only for heart disease, but for other health problems, including obesity, type 2 diabetes, gastrointestinal disorders, osteoporosis, and insomnia. Finally, this knowledge is put to work, as Dr. Goodman offers clear guidelines on how to select and use magnesium supplements to greatest effect.

Many drugs are designed to relieve the symptoms of heart disease, but none of them eliminates the root cause of the problem. In *Magnificent Magnesium,* you will discover how a simple all-natural mineral can improve the function of your heart and help you regain control of your health.

$14.95 US • 192 pages • 6 x 9-inch quality paperback • ISBN 978-0-7570-0391-2

For more information about our books, visit our website at www.squareonepublishers.com